Genetics and the Quality of Life

Genetics and the Quality of Life

edited by
Charles Birch
and
Paul Abrecht

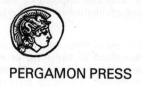

PERGAMON PRESS

Pergamon Press (Australia) Pty Limited, P.O. Box 544, Potts Point, NSW, 2011
Pergamon Press Ltd, Headington Hill Hall, Oxford OX3 OBW
Pergamon Press Inc., Fairview Park, Elmsford, NY 10523

First published 1975

© 1975 Charles Birch on behalf of World Council of Churches, Geneva

Printed in Singapore by Toppan Printing Co (S) Pte Ltd

National Library of Australia Cataloguing-in-Publication entry:
Genetics and the quality of life: [papers of a symposium]/
    edited by Charles Birch [and] Paul Abrecht.
    —Rushcutters Bay, N.S.W.: Pergamon Press, 1975
    Index.
    Symposium held in Zurich, Sw., 1973.
    Includes bibliographies.
    ISBN 0 08 018210 0.
    ISBN 0 08 019861 9 Paperback.

    1. Genetics—Experiments—Moral and religious aspects—
    Congresses. I. Birch, Charles, ed. II Abrecht, Paul,
    joint ed.

    174.9574

Contents

v

Grateful acknowledgement is made to
Annette Robinson and Annette Halcomb
for their meticulous and painstaking
work in seeing this work through
to publication.

PART I

Introduction

This volume contains the papers and the report of a consultation on Genetics and the Quality of Life, in Zurich, 25-29 June 1973, organized by the sub-unit on Church and Society of the World Council of Churches in cooperation with the Christian Medical Commission. It was attended by thirty-five persons including clinical geneticists, population geneticists, immuno-geneticists, reproductive biologists, pediatricians, psychiatrists, physicians, obstetricians, ethicists, theologians, social workers, lawyers, legislators and politicians. The group was unique compared with other groups drawn together for similar purposes by representing many different social and geographical perspectives, and by being ecumenical in character, including as it did Protestants, Orthodox and Roman Catholics of widely differing views, as well as some with no particular religious commitment. A list of participants is included at the end of the volume.

Ecumenical interest in the ethical issues resulting from developments in the biological sciences first arose at a conference on *Technology, Faith, and the Future of Man* in Geneva, July 1970. In June 1971, the Working Committee on Church and Society, meeting in Nemi, Italy, decided to undertake 'a pilot study in some very specific areas of scientific activity which generate disturbing problems'. The field of genetics was chosen, not because the issues raised are essentially different from those raised by other technologies, but because they are immediately recognizable by men and women everywhere as important for their marriages, for their children's future as well as for the future of the human race, and because these issues touch on many deep-rooted religious and cultural attitudes.

The specific genetic problem chosen had to do with the ethical questions that arise from the application of modern methods for detecting and reducing the incidence of genetic disease in the community. The Nemi meeting therefore recommended that 'the World Council of Churches establish a panel consisting primarily of geneticists and theologians' to advise it and its member churches on fundamental questions of genetic counselling, foetal diagnosis and abortion, and genetic correction.

The recommendation was placed before the Executive Committee of the World Council of Churches at its meeting in Sofia, Bulgaria (5-9 September 1971), and before the meeting of the Central Committee of the Council in Utrecht, August 1972. In approving the plan for a panel the Central Committee noted:

'The Committee accepts the terms of reference outlined for this panel, without necessarily endorsing all the assumptions of the document by the

Working Committee. The Committee emphasizes the importance of having on the panel geneticists with a broad understanding of the social responsibility of their science and sensitivity to Christian conceptions of life; the panel should also include theologians, ethicists and other church members concerned with the human, social and spiritual issues at stake in such experiments of genetic correction.'
(Minutes of the Central Committee of the World Council of Churches, Utrecht, August 1972, pp. 43-44.)

In preparation for the meeting in Zurich, nineteen of the participants prepared papers on one of five topics:
• Ethical and Psychiatric Problems of Genetic Counselling
• Social and Ethical Problems in Caring for Genetically Handicapped Children
• Political and Social Issues in the Public Discussion of the Prevention of Genetic Defects
• Ethical Problems in Foetal Diagnosis and Abortion
• Ethical and Cultural Problems Raised by Eugenics.
Most of these papers were circulated in advance of the meeting and were discussed in two days of plenary sessions under the chairmanship of Professor Charles Birch (Australia).

The panel then divided into three Working Groups for drafting the report and conclusions:
Genetic Counselling
    Chairman: Fr. Paul Verghese (India)
    Vice-Chairman: Prof. R. Murray (USA)
Foetal Diagnosis and Selective Abortion
    Chairman: Prof. Roger Shinn (USA)
    Vice-Chairman: Prof. A. E. Boyo (Nigeria)
Political, Social and Ethical Implications of Eugenic Programmes
    Chairman: Prof. Bentley Glass (USA)
    Vice-Chairman: Dr R. G. Edwards (UK)
The panel reassembled in plenary on the final day to review the draft reports. These reports as amended and revised in plenary session were committed to a drafting committee who produced the present integrated report and findings based on the material of the Working Groups.

The panel restricted its considerations to genetic procedures now in practice or about to be practised. It deliberately did not deal with highly speculative proposals such as cloning and 'positive genetics'. The purpose of this restriction was to establish ethical guidelines where most needed now, and to examine a number of specific areas of concern where examination might serve as models for more extensive studies.

As far as possible technical terms have been avoided, but where this has not been possible the terms used are defined in a glossary appended at the end of the document.

Clearly this report is not the final word on the issues posed. Indeed the panel was conscious throughout that it was wrestling with some questions on which there could be generally no clear ethical guidance and on which opinions within the panel itself differed greatly. Nevertheless, a great deal of unanimity was achieved and so the findings of the consultation do mark an advance in presenting some guide lines for the future.

Charles Birch
Paul Abrecht

PART II

Ethical and Political Issues
Raised by Genetics

CHAPTER 1

Genetics and moral responsibility

Charles Birch

School of Biological Sciences, University of Sydney, Australia

Each new power won *by* man is a power *over* man as well.
C. S. Lewis (1965)

The inequality of man is a consequence of genetic and environmental differences. We have tended to believe that whereas a lot could be done about reducing environmental inequality, little if anything could be done about reducing genetic inequality. The situation is now different.

This decade has brought advances in genetics that make possible the practice of certain eugenic programmes hitherto impossible. Negative eugenics, the elimination or reduction of deleterious genes, now has practicable programmes operating in many countries. Positive genetics, procedures to increase 'desirable' genes, has hypothetical programmes which may, within a few years, become practicable.

The objective of negative eugenics, to reduce the incidence of genetic disease, is a rational and laudable one. It can be regarded as an extension by man of what happens without his intervention already. One out of every 130 conceptions ends before the mother realizes she is pregnant because the fertilized egg (probably defective) never attaches itself to the uterus. Some 25 per cent of all conceptions fail to survive to birth and of these a third have identifiable chromosomal abnormalities. Of those that are born, three out of every 100 have some genetic defect.

The hypothetical schemes for 'improving' the genetic constitution of man by positive eugenics, selective breeding and other means, is much more debatable. There is the objection of incursion into human freedom and the dilemma as to which qualities to breed for (Kass 1971). Gene therapy may soon be practicable to ameliorate some genetic diseases but as yet advances are not such as to warrant its use on human patients (Friedmann and Roblin 1972). Concerning positive eugenics and the future, Lerner (1968) has said, 'Clearly, whatever biological problems the wonders of euphenics and genetical engineering may solve, they will create many unprecedented social and ethical problems, for the solution of which much collective wisdom will be needed. The requisite wisdom is unlikely to come from the genetical engineers alone, because it involves moral issues on which they are not experts. The traditional ethical guidelines have come from religion, but the new religion of science and technology that is arising, with its hierachy of scientists instead of priests, with its sacred language of mathematics instead of Latin, with its sacrifices of traffic casualties instead of heretics, and with space exploration for its Crusades, is as yet not capable of providing any.' These words of wisdom are as applicable to the problems of negative eugenics which are already with us and which therefore have an urgency greater than is the case with positive eugenics. The medical profession has already accepted major responsibility in the issues of negative genetics but this profession has both evolved and is organized in a way that tends not to equip it for handling these responsibilities. Nor are the various community and counselling services of churches and other organizations ready to deal with these urgent problems.

Genetically determined debility versus socially determined debility
Before proceeding to consider the sorts of moral responsibilities that negative eugenics presents to us, there is a prior issue to consider. There are those who, while recognizing the ethical problems raised by eugenics, nevertheless consider these to be quite unimportant matters for man's attention at present. There are two sorts of argument for this view.

(1) The problems raised by the 'quantity' of people in the world are far more urgent than those to do with the genetical 'quality' of people. It is the population explosion, not the fact that a small proportion of people have genetic diseases, that should be engaging our attention. If it were possible to quantify human suffering, the human suffering caused by over-population would be seen to dominate the scene in most places in the world. Moreover, besides the quantity of people there are other major contributory causes to human misery that rank much higher than genetic disease. Factors such as poverty, malnutrition and social deprivation have a variety of causes in addition to over-population.

The vast majority of people are born with a 'normal' complement of genes. They are normal genetically, but their genes are never given a chance because of sub-optimal environments they live in. According to a report of one United Nations agency, 100 million children in the world today will grow up without a chance of becoming normal healthy people. These are the poor, underprivileged, overpopulated and hungry children of one-third of the world whose families have to live on less than $200 a year. In many developing countries 50 per cent of the children who reach the age of one year will be dead by the age of five years from infection superimposed on malnutrition. In the developing countries as a whole the population/doctor ratio in the capital cities may be less than 1,000:1 and in the rural areas and slums it is often 10,000:1 and can even exceed 100,000:1. This, itself, is largely a product of inflicting western style medical education and practice on countries with quite different needs.

The chief and overwhelming ethical and moral issue facing us is that the organization of our world is such that it guarantees that a large fraction of human beings will be the victims of the environment they were born into with little chance of rising above it. What we have to fight for primarily is the liberation of the gene; to give our genes a chance, these genes of all people everywhere that are held in straitjackets that are primarily non-genetic.

Is it not a matter of rather low priority to spend time and effort on the problems that concern a small segment of mankind, namely those with genetic defects? Lewontin (1971) chided those of his genetical colleagues whom he considered to be preoccupied with ethical problems arising out of the application of eugenics. 'We are told that if we can diagnose genetical disorders *in utero,* a serious ethical problem arises in the decision to deprive a possibly debilitated foetus of its right to life. In a more futuristic vein, we are asked to ponder the weighty ethical problem that arises if we could manipulate an individual's genes at birth or before, since we would be making a decision about a person's biological nature and the biological nature of future generations . . . What is seldom realized is that the preoccupation with individual moral issues such as these, however serious they may be, is the result of a class bias peculiar to scientists, academics and other middle class persons. For such privileged persons for whom personal freedom and choice are taken for granted, these individual interferences with liberty and destiny seem fraught with significance. But they are uttered blind to the fact that large groups of human beings are victims, by *socially determined* necessity, of scientific decisions and research priorities.' Lewontin was not arguing against genetic screening programmes that might alleviate suffering in black ghettos. He was arguing against an elitist concern about genetical manipulation and its ethical problems whilst ignoring the fact that, for a majority of the people in the world, social and political circumstances prevent them from having a chance in life. The social and ethical problems of our time are not primarily those caused by wrong genetics but by wrong social and political systems. That is a fact which is hardly disputable. It is of course extremely difficult to assess the relative importance of genes and environment in determining inequalities between individuals, especially in such characteristics as cognitive skill. Recent studies of Jencks *et al.* (1972) suggest that genes explain about 45 per cent of the variation in cognitive skills of Americans, with environment explaining about 35 per cent. The tendency of environmentally advantaged families to have genetically advantaged children explains the remaining 20 per cent. This is because economically successful adults may have been successful as a result of having more than their share of favourable genes that lead to high cognitive skills. Those who started life with genetic advantages tend to get environmental advantages as well. This exacerbates inequality and is, in Jencks' view, a reason for some of the major difficulties in social engineering aimed to reduce inequality. Be that as it may, the most immediate alleviation of inequality in many communities will be achieved by social engineering rather than genetic manipulation.

However, because one path of reform may produce more immediate effects than another is not a sound reason for paying no attention to the other. It is a reason for putting the weight of effort into the more important problem. Indeed, if our efforts were more rationally planned we might make a priority list of major problems as Platt (1969) tried to do in his widely quoted article entitled 'What we must do'. He happened to rate the threat of total annihilation by nuclear warfare as the top problem. By that rating he did not imply that we should all put our effort exclusively into trying to resolve that problem. We should no doubt all put an effort into it, but not exclusively. Moreover, the choice before us is not simply whether to proceed with quantity control or quality control of human populations. An acceptable quantity control is birth control aimed toward limitation and spacing of children. Quantity control encourages the two child replacement family. Those precious two should be of the highest quality, hence the desirability for quality control to go hand in hand with population control. The two can be done together.

(2) In developing countries, where infant mortality is high, deaths and illness due to genetic defects constitute a small proportion of the total illness and deaths. It is only when total infant mortality declines that deaths and illness caused by genetic defects are considered to assume a public health problem. So it has been argued that the pressing problems of developing countries do not include the relatively small contribution to human suffering made by congenital disease. However, Lappé (1972) has indicated that this may well be a short-sighted point of view. The incidence may be higher than in developed countries, the interaction between environment and expression of genetic defects may

be different, the spectrum of genetic diseases may be different in tropical countries, and because care and treatment for congenitally handicapped are less developed in these countries, the amount of suffering may be higher. Lappé gives some evidence to indicate that each of these points may well be valid ones. He points out, for example, the now well-known fact that as many as one in 64 children amongst West African blacks have sickle cell anaemia compared with one in 484 blacks in the United States of America. The proportion is even higher in Central Africa with some 4 per cent of babies having sickle cell anaemia. The high incidence is associated with the resistance to malaria of those individuals who are heterozygous, that is they contain a normal gene alongside the sickle cell gene. Currently infant mortality there is around 60 per cent to 70 per cent. When this is brought down to 10 per cent, perhaps in a few years following improved public health programmes, then the 4 per cent deaths from sickle cell anaemia will be very significant.

The case for being concerned
The case for being seriously concerned about our moral responsibilities for suffering caused by genetic disease is that more than 1,600 human diseases caused by genetic defects have been identified (Friedmann 1971). Whilst some are very rare, others, such as cystic fibrosis and sickle cell anaemia are relatively common diseases. About half of all cases of congenital blindness and about half of all cases of congenital deafness are due to defective genes. Dobzhansky (1970) has warned against underestimating 'the magnitude of the problem of genetically conditioned ill-health and inborn defects and abnormalities'. He refers to the following figures for Northern Ireland: 'at least 4 per cent of the infants are born with genetic defects which will incapacitate them more or less seriously at some time during their lives. This is in addition to abortions and stillbirths, which occur in about 14 per cent of recorded pregnancies, an unknown but substantial fraction of the abortions and stillbirths are genetic. About 26 per cent of hospital beds in Northern Ireland were occupied by persons with genetically caused defects, about 6 per cent of consultations with general practitioners and 8 per cent with medical specialists involved such persons. This is a great deal of human misery.' Further, this burden of genetic defects is growing heavier, allegedly because modern medicine enables the defective persons to live longer and pass on their genes to the next generation. We have a twofold problem, present suffering and future increase of genetic diseases and therefore even greater human suffering.

The most frequently occurring genetic defects are due to deleterious genes that have a large effect. Carter (1972) estimated that in European populations this is about ten per 1,000 live births, which is twice that for abnormalities in the chromosomes, the second major group of genetic diseases. In an appendix to his book, Dorfman (1972) has a list of forty-two diseases due to genes that have a large effect; in twenty-seven of them prenatal diagnosis is possible and in fifteen of them he considers prenatal diagnosis to be potentially possible. Diagnosis leads to the possibility of selective abortion.

A second group of genetic defects are due to chromosomal abnormalities which occur in five out of every 1,000 births. This risk increases with the age of the mother. *Table 1.1* shows the results of a study of 4,500 consecutively born infants in New Haven (Lubs and Ruddle 1970).

Table 1.1

The risk of having a chromosomally abnormal child

Age of mother	Number per birth	Per cent risk
10–14	0/19	—
15–19	1/490	0.20
20–24	8/1531	0.52
25–29	4/1423	0.28
30–34	1/635	0.16
35–39	4/277	1.44
40–44	1/62	1.61
45–49	0/3	—
Total	22/4469	

In this study 1.5 per cent of all children born to mothers thirty-five and over were chromosomally abnormal, such abnormalities causing relatively mild to extremely serious symptoms.

The most important genetic defect for which genetic screening can be done at present is Down's syndrome (Mongolism), both because of the severity of the condition, 95 per cent severely retarded and 5 per cent mentally retarded and because of its prevalence, about one in 600 live births. Down's syndrome is due to one too many chromosomes, a total of forty-seven instead of the normal human complement of forty-six; one of the chromosomes is present in triplicate instead of the normal duplicate. The risk of having a live-born child with Down's syndrome to women over forty is about one in one hundred. Children with Down's syndrome comprise between a third and a quarter of all children with severe mental handicap at school age (Carter 1972). Four thousand infants with Down's syndrome are born each year in the United States. Lifetime institutional care for each one costs about 250,000 dollars. Friedmann (1971) has estimated that if all pregnancies in women thirty-five years of age or older were subject to detection for Down's syndrome, the rate of occurrence of the disease would be reduced by half the present level if selective abortion were practised. In the state of New South Wales in Australia about half of the annual births with Down's syndrome (sixty out of 120 per year) will survive to enter an average of thirty years of institutional life. On current costs this amounts to $A5,000 per year which is $A9 million for each cohort of survivors, not allowing for increasing costs of institutionalism, (Charles Kerr— personal communication).

After Down's syndrome the next most frequent genetic defects in live births due to abnormal chromosome number are abnormal numbers of sex chromosomes—XXX, XXY and XYY, instead of the normal XY male or XX female. Each of these defects has a frequency of the order of one in 1,000 live births. The handicap with these is less than with Down's syndrome (Carter 1972).

Amongst the metabolic diseases due to deleterious genes that have a large effect, there is a tremendous range in incidence of the different diseases and in severity of the symptoms from one disease to another. Inherited deficiency in the activity of the enzyme glucose-6-phosphate dehydrogenase is world wide. This is a potentially lethal disorder resulting in haemolytic anaemia. It is present in 14 per cent of black men and 2 per cent of black women in the United States. In Southeast Asia it is the commonest cause of potentially brain damaging neonatal jaundice (Charles Kerr—personal communication). For this disease screening is now possible.

Cystic fibrosis is a genetic disease present in one in 2,500 live births. Symptoms are recurrent pulmonary infection and failure of the child to thrive. Screening is potentially possible. One in 25 Europeans and North Americans are carriers (heterozygous) for this defective gene. If they could be identified, as we may well anticipate will become possible, then marriage partners would be able to know the chance of their children being defective and could then take appropriate steps to avoid having defective children.

One in 10,000 live births in the USA have the genetic disease phenylketonuria (PKU). This amounts to 200-300 cases each year. In this disease the liver is unable to manufacture an essential enzyme. The effects are severe mental retardation. If diagnosed at birth, by bio-chemical tests, treatment is possible to reduce the serious effects of the disorder. Almost all states in the USA have laws making screening for PKU mandatory at birth. Costs of screening programmes far outweigh the costs of institutionalizing cases undiagnozed in early life. The situation however is not quite so straightforward for not every child with a positive test for phenylketonuria develops the mental retardation usually associated with the untreated disease.

Sickle cell anaemia is a debilitating genetic disease. Many of those affected die before they are twenty years old and few live beyond forty years of age. In the USA it occurs in one in 500 black children. A total of between 25,000 and 50,000 people have the disease and another two million carry the trait (Culliton 1972a, 1972b). The incidence of the disease is higher elsewhere; for example, one in 64 children of West African blacks are affected. The disease almost exclusively affects black people. Screening programmes can identify carriers, but as yet there is no satisfactory method of identifying the disease in the foetus. A multi-million dollar screening programme in the USA has already raised a great number of ethical and social problems which are receiving attention from ethicists and clinical geneticists.

Tay-Sachs disease is also caused by a recessive gene when present in double dose. It has again a one in four chance of appearing in children of carrier parents. Carriers can be identified as can the affected foetus. The incidence of the disease is high in certain ethnic groups and could be completely eliminated by screening and abortion of defective foetuses. It occurs in one in 900 births among marriages between Ashkenaz Jews in the United States. It is estimated that the three million Jewish Americans under thirty years of age will produce thirty-three cases of Tay Sachs disease annually. Tay-Sachs disease is the infantile form of amaurotic idiocy. It results in complete mental degeneration and blindness and death usually before the age of three or four years. The total cost of carrier detection, prenatal diagnosis and termination of pregnancy of risk cases for all Jewish individuals in the USA who are under thirty has been estimated to be nearly six million dollars. The total hospital costs for the 990 cases of Tay-Sachs disease these individuals would produce over a thirty year period is about thirty-five million dollars (Harris 1972).

Reducing the burden
What can be done now about reducing the incidence of genetic diseases? Quite a lot. It is, as has already been indicated, possible to identify some of these diseases in the affected foetus by means of the technique amniocentesis. Selective abortion may then be practised (for example for Down's syndrome). Secondly, for an increasing number of genetic diseases the 'heterozygous' carriers of the defective genes, though themselves normal, can be identified by appropriate biochemical tests, or in the case of chromosome abnormalities, by chromosome analysis. The list of genetic diseases for which the heterozygous carriers can be

detected increases at the rate of three or more each year (Glass 1972), with over 300 already that can be detected. It is thus possible to identify the critical marriages, in which two carriers are wed, by appropriate screening programmes. There is no justification in avoiding this responsibility in areas of high incidence of genetic disease, for example, Mediterranean anaemia (thalassemia) in Mediterranean peoples, Tay-Sachs disease in Jewish Americans in New York, porphyria in the Afrikaner population in South Africa and phenylketonuria, which can be identified at birth, almost everywhere.

When something is known of genetical diseases in family histories it becomes feasible to screen suspected carriers of the defective gene. For example, the female carriers of haemophilia and the Duchenne type of muscular dystrophy can be detected by appropriate tests. The sons of such women have a fifty-fifty chance of being affected. Since sexing of the foetus *in utero* is now possible, abortion can be offered if the parents are unwilling to take the high risk of having a male child. In such cases the parents have a fifty-fifty chance of aborting a normal male. Conversely, if a male haemophiliac married, he might wish for a female child to be aborted, since these would be carriers whereas his sons would all be normal. The objective of screening heterozygotes is to reduce the number of children born with a particular disease. Such a programme may be effective in this objective but that is not to say that it will be very effective in reducing the incidence of the deleterious recessive gene in the community. The eugenic programme would have to be extremely severe (for example, no reproduction of heterozygotes) to greatly reduce the incidence of the gene. Some programmes may achieve a considerable reduction in this direction. However, it is totally unrealistic to imagine that eventually negative eugenic programmes would eliminate deleterious recessive genes. Most of us carry, on the average, several of them. If we were to eliminate all of them we would eliminate mankind in the process (Lerner 1968).

What are the benefits to be gained from these procedures of negative eugenics? The immediate and most important one is reduction in suffering. A second benefit is reduction in cost to the community. Consider chromosomal defects alone. Lubs and Lubs (1972) have estimated that in 1967 in the USA 300,000 infants were born to mothers thirty-five years of age and older. This constitutes 10 per cent of all births. At a cost of $15 million this group of pregnancies could have been screened. Assuming that 1.5 per cent of births were chromosomally abnormal some 4,500 chromosomally defective children would have been born to these mothers. If the costs in special medical care and education may be conservatively put at $2,000 per year, these special costs over twenty years would be 180 million dollars.

Ethical problems

Along with the developments of negative eugenics come a host of ethical problems. Murray (1972) lists the following questions that he considers should be answered before effective genetic screening programmes are instituted. Who is to be tested? Should testing be voluntary or compulsory? What should be done with information obtained from testing? What will be the attitude of the public and their peers towards the individual who is identified as a carrier? In relation to these sorts of questions Lappé et al. (1972); Macintyre (1972); Hilton et al. (1972) and others have suggested a number of guide lines which are considered to be imperative, such as pre- and post-counselling by expert members of a panel who control input to the diagnostic laboratories. Decision making that is left to individual doctors can lead to error, personal anxiety and confusion, and abuse of expensive resources. Even when firm guide lines are followed, risk still remains of misuse of genetic information derived from screening. It is becoming clearer with more experience that the rights and respect of the individual can be very easily abused if screening programmes are not preceded by a careful anticipation in great detail of the ethical and social problems that can arise.

The issues raised by amniocentesis primarily centre upon abortion following detection. (1) How serious must the defect be to warrant abortion for those who are prepared to proceed this way? Alongside the deleterious defects there is still, in Down's syndrome for example, the capacity for performing a variety of human activities such as being affectionate and responsive to affection. The negative has in some way to be balanced with the positive. (2) What is the attitude to abortion in cases where some remedial treatment is available to the child who is born defective? Some will argue for the prevention of birth of the defective child.

Others will argue for treatment even though such treatment may have uncertain effects. Probably most would argue for the continuation of efforts to find ways of treating such illness rather than to rely entirely on detection and abortion. Bentley Glass (1972) considers that the ethical question of abortion is more acute in the case of a simple dominant gene of malignant character such as that which produces retino-blastoma, a condition that is invariably fatal in childhood. Surgical removal of the cancerous condition often has excellent results permitting the child to retain one eye and to grow to normal adulthood. Since most of these patients then marry they will pass on the severe genetic disorder to half of their children who will also require the radical surgery. Should they remain childless? If they do not the frequency of the disease will inevitably rise in future generations. How do you measure what might seem a present value against future disvalue of this sort?

Professor C. H. Waddington, of the Institute of Genetics in Edinburgh, put his view quite bluntly once when he said 'If I deliberately cripple a child, I am a monster and the community will lock me up. If a government lined up 1,000 babies against a wall and shot them, a political bloodbath would follow. But what if I knowingly take a one in four risk of conceiving a crippled child? Or kill a child while driving when drunk? Am I a victim of bad luck, to be sympathized with—or a gambler whose rashness is too cruel to be tolerated?' Those who argue against abortion of seriously defective foetuses might also be asked their attitude to preventing (say by a drug) the spontaneous abortions that now occur. If this were done it could involve an enormous increase in the number of children born mentally defective since the great majority of chromosomally abnormal foetuses are spontaneously aborted (Clarke 1969).

Genetic inequality and moral responsibility

Genetics confronts us with the inequality of man which is the human predicament. No two individuals, except they be identical twins, have the same genetic endowment. All men are different. Some are endowed with the capacity for developing many talents, others have a few. Still others are burdened with serious genetic defects that incapacitate them for life. What then is our attitude to this unequal distribution of the goods and the bads in our genetic endowment?

If I am more or less normal, it is through no merit of my own. That others have genetic deficiencies is no fault of theirs. The mongol child could have been me. The fact that others have not, through no fault of theirs, changes for me the character of my having. It drives me to a realization of both the unity of mankind and the cost of creation. All are called to share the cost. The genetic inequality of man makes me realize my responsibility to mankind. Through chance some must suffer more than others. How can I make their suffering less? A community becomes responsible for the cost of creation, the misfits and incapacitated, through every responsible member of that community. This is the high meaning of justice. Justice does not require equality but, as Rawls (1972) has pleaded with eloquence, it does require that men share one another's fate.

There seem to be two ways in which I can share the genetic burden of mankind. I can reduce the total burden. And I can share the burden by helping to alleviate the suffering, be it of the maimed or of their families. I can reduce the burden when, with others, I seek to reduce the number of people who are born genetically maimed. If I am a parent I have that direct responsibility to my children. The community has its responsibility in making the choices open to parents clear to them. That involves accurate and sympathetic counselling about specific genetical diseases. It also involves the development of a sense of high obligation. Sir Alan Parkes (1969) in discussing 'The right to reproduce in an overcrowded world' drew up a 'Declaration of Human Obligations' that ran:

It is an obligation of men and women

(a) Not to produce unwanted children.

(b) Not to take a substantial risk of begetting a mentally or physically defective child.

(c) Not to produce children, because of irresponsibility or religious observance, merely as a by-product of sexual intercourse.

(d) To plan the number and spacing of births in the best interests of mother, child and the rest of the family.

(e) To give the best possible mental and physical environment to the child during its most formative years and to produce children, therefore, only in the course of an affectionate and stable relationship between man and woman.

(f) However convinced the individual may be of his or her superior qualities, not for this reason to produce children of numbers which, if equalled by everyone, would be demographically catastrophic.

In commenting on his 'Declaration' Parkes regarded clause (e) as a counsel of perfection and one to be aimed at. Clause (f) seems to present difficulties to some people who like to believe that superiority lies in their family line. However, Parkes points out that so far as we know the great reservoir of human talent lies in the genetic pool held by ordinary people.

Who decides?

Should this important area of life be left entirely to individual decisions albeit decisions that have been open to educational influences? The idea that the state should enter into this kind of weighing up process for the social good is widely accepted in other areas of life. Genetic defects cause a huge amount of suffering in the world. Is it not a crime if even a single individual suffers unnecessarily? Should not the state be involved in some way?

An exploratory conference of the World Council of Churches on these and other problems held in 1970 (Gill 1970) agreed that the new sorts of ethical judgments raised by biological discoveries forces upon us the need to reconsider the relationship between individual freedom to make decisions and the need for society to make decisions which will limit the area within which individuals are free to decide. Society of course always limits individual freedom of choice to some extent. The conference raised the question as to whether we are to be more self-conscious about this and plan the way society limits or permits the individual's freedom of choice. Thus, however shocking it is to our present ideas of human (individual) freedom, can we allow individuals to have complete freedom in their choice of family size (when any more than two children per family adds to the world's population explosion), or their choice of sex of offspring (when that becomes possible)? And can we allow freedom of choice where there is a risk of producing genetically defective children?

Christian ethics have traditionally been addressed to individuals making moral decisions. How do we work out an ethic which is appropriate to the shaping of society and institutions in such a way that mankind will survive and individuals will have a chance to exercise appropriate freedom? That, broadly stated, is the ethical dilemma that confronts us and will increasingly confront us as biology adds to its discoveries about how to control both the quantity and the quality of life.

Acknowledgments

I gratefully acknowledge helpful criticism and comment on the manuscript from Professor Sir Macfarlane Burnet, School of Microbiology, University of Melbourne; Professor Charles Kerr, Department of Preventive and Social Medicine, University of Sydney; Professor Michael Lerner, Genetics Department, University of California, Berkeley; and Professor R. J. Walsh, Dean, Faculty of Medicine, University of New South Wales.

References
CARTER, C. O. (1972) Practical aspects of early diagnosis. *In* Harris, Maureen (ed.) See below.
CLARKE, C. A. (1969) Problems raised by developments in genetics. *In* Ebling, F. J. (ed.) *Biology and Ethics.* p.93. (Academic Press: London.)
CULLITON, B. J. (1972*a*) Sickle cell anemia: the route from obscurity to prominence. *Science.* **178**, 138.
—(1972*b*) Sickle cell anemia: national program raises problems as well as hopes. *Science.* **178**, 283.
DOBZHANSKY, Th. (1970) Human evolution and ethical issues. (Un-

published address to US Conference for the World Council of Churches: Buck-Hill Falls, Pa. April 1970.)

DORFMAN, A. (ed.) (1972) *Antenatal Diagnosis.* (The University of Chicago Press.)

FRIEDMANN, T. (1971) Prenatal diagnosis of genetic disease. *Scientific American.* **225:5,** 34.

FRIEDMANN, T. & ROBLIN, R. (1972) Gene therapy for human genetic disease. *Science.* **175,** 949.

GILL, D. M. (1970) *From Here to Where? Technology, Faith and the Future of Man.* (World Council of Churches: Geneva.)

GLASS, Bentley (1972) Human heredity and ethical problems. *Perspectives in Biology and Medicine.* **15,** 237.

HARRIS, Maureen (ed.) (1972) *Ethical Problems in Human Genetics: Early Diagnosis of Genetic Defects.* Fogarty International Center Publication Proceedings No. 6, DHEW Pub. No. (NIH) 72-75. p. 64. (National Technical Information Service, US Dept. of Commerce.)

HILTON, B., CALLAHAN, D., HARRIS, Maureen, CONDLIFFE, P. & BERKLEY, B. (eds.) (1973) *Ethical Issues in Human Genetics: Genetic Counseling and the Use of Genetic Knowledge.* Fogarty International Center Publication Proceedings No. 13. (Plenum Publishing Corp.: New York.)

JENCKS, C., SMITH, M., ACLAND, H., BANE, M. J., COHEN, D., HEYNS, B. & MICHELSON, S. (1972) *Inequality: A Reassessment of the Effect of Family and Schooling in America.* (Basic Books: New York.)

KASS, L. R. (1971) The new biology: what price relieving man's estate? *Science.* **174,** 779.

LAPPE, M. A. (1972) Problems of congenital disease and abnormalities in the developing countries. (Unpublished.)

LAPPE, M. A., GOSTAFSON, J. M. & ROBLIN, R. (1972) Ethical and social issues in screening for genetic disease. *New England Journal of Medicine.* **286,** 1129.

LERNER, I. M. (1968) *Heredity, Evolution and Society.* p. 179. (W. H. Freeman: San Francisco.)

LEWIS, C. S. (1965) *The Abolition of Man.* p. 70. (Macmillan: New York.)

LEWONTIN, R. C. (1971) Science and ethics. *Bioscience.* **21,** 799.

LUBS, H. A. & LUBS, M. L. E. (1972) Indications for amniocentesis. *In* Dorfman, A. (ed.). See above, p. 17.

LUBS, H. A. & RUDDLE, F. H. (1970) Chromosomal abnormalities in the human population: estimation of rates based on New Haven newborn study. *Science.* **169,** 1195.

MACINTYRE, M. N. (1972) Counseling in cases inviting antenatal diagnosis. *In* Dorfman, A. (ed.). See above. p. 63.

MURRAY, R. F. (1972) Problems behind the promise: ethical issues in mass genetic screening. *Hastings Center Report.* **2:2,** 11.

PARKES, A. S. (1969) The right to reproduce in an overcrowded world. *In* Ebling, F. J. (ed.) *Biology and Ethics.* p. 109. (Academic Press: London.)

PLATT, J. (1969) What we must do. *Science,* **166,** 1115.

RAWLS, H. (1972) *A Theory of Justice.* (Harvard University Press: Cambridge, Massachusetts.)

CHAPTER 2

Ethics and the new biology

I. Michael Lerner

*Department of Genetics and
Institute of Personality Assessment and Research,
University of California, Berkeley, California, USA*

Genetics, or more broadly, evolution covers three domains of thought. Firstly, there is the *mode* of thought or the outlook. This includes, for instance, the idea of historicity of the past and of continuity of change. Though the Greek philosophers knew all this, it was Darwin and Marx who really brought the outlook into the open in terms of human society. It was also Darwinism that produced rejection of anthropocentrism, the idea that man was the centre of the universe. From the historical stand-point Darwin was, of course, right: in cosmic history man was not the centre either of the universe or of our galaxy, or of the solar system, or of this planet. The quaint concept that man was created in the image of his Maker led, of course, to lip service to the concept of theocentrism while assuming, in practice, anthropocentrism. The Darwinian rejection was scientifically and sociologically a healthy thing. But today, I wonder if we should not return to anthropocentrism. We *have* become the centre if not of the universe, then, perhaps, of our galaxy, and certainly of Earth. Are not in reality our highest-minded efforts, whether it is in the fight against hunger and disease or in preservation of resources and of natural beauty, addressed primarily to the satisfaction of human wants? Are not our alleged obligations to other species really hedonistic in origin? Why should we kid ourselves?

Another aspect of our mode of thought is also a scientific reversal. It refers to the formulation of questions which concern those of us with intellectual curiosity. Francis Crick, for instance, suggested that the important questions are 'What are we?', 'Why are we here?', 'Why does the world work in this particular way?' This is another turnabout! Modern science was made possible by Galileo's substitution of 'how' for 'why'. And now we have one of the great champions of reductionism,

---

* A lecture originally given to students in the Population Biology course at Stanford University in 1973 and presented with little alteration to this consultation.

that is in the ultimate a mechanistic type of explaining nature, asking 'why' questions!

The second domain of thought is that of *technical application*. I do not need to specify the significance of genetics in medicine, nutrition, public health, mental health, agriculture, quality of environment and so forth. I am sure that you have already heard enough about the forthcoming marvels of gene therapy or of organ transplants and need no convincing.

Finally we must deal with *ethical and moral issues* which the developments in the new biology have raised. I do not care to debate whether genetical engineering is a quantum jump or merely an extension of what for centuries was called medicine, or whether the possibilities of physical or chemical manipulation of behaviour provides a discontinuity in the history of educational practice. I don't think that this is terribly important. Whether or not we deal with threshold phenomena, we do have some problems in having to reformulate attitudes or definitions of our goals and in having to find guidelines for social behaviour. The problem by no means is one of genetics.

Breakdown of values

Fifteen years ago, the anthropologist Clyde Kluckhohn without any reference to DNA clearly saw that: 'We lack a system of general ideas and values to give meaning to human life in the mid-twentieth century'. Others, like the physicist-philosopher Max Born have concluded in despair that it is modern science that bears responsibility for the breakdown of ethical values. And this, incidentally, in the face of the rising counter-culture; in which anti-intellectualism, occultism, astrology, scientology, satanism, mysticism, cults of psychotherapeutic techniques, each more bizarre than the previously fashionable one, emphasis on psychedelic experience and even glossolalia; seem to become ever more pervading. But just to place things into perspective, I must say that I realize that there is little reason to wax hysterical about urgencies or priorities simply because solutions, should there be any, are not readily at hand. Indeed, I realize that man has ever been facing immediately pressing problems. For instance, here is a quotation: 'You must know that the world has grown old and does not remain in its former vigour. It bears witness to its own decline. The rainfall and the sun's warmth are both diminishing; the metals are nearly exhausted; the husbandman is failing in the fields.' This is not Paul Ehrlich. It was written in about A.D. 260 by St. Cyprian, one of the Fathers of the Church.

Before getting down to cases, I want to say a few words about the general debate going on regarding the nature and basis for ethical guidelines which might be used to seek answers to the issues posed by the explosion of knowledge, in this age of scientific techniques if not of scientific attitudes.

I believe it should be emphasized that there is absolutely no agreement even in the area of what is called metaethics, that is the branch of epistemology which deals with the criteria of validation of statements about what is right or wrong. There are many varieties of theories in this very fundamental field. Thus, the relativist ones assume that judgments vary from group to group or even from individual to individual. Theories arising from logical positivism say that only preferences rather than statements of generalized judgments are meaningful. Many others are absolutist, deriving from diverse bases, such as supernatural, rationalist, empirical and so on.

Whatever the case may be, any number of ethical systems for this age of technology have been proposed. One claims that it is possible to derive a rationalistic objective ethical system from the second law of thermodynamics. Others have used as touchstones of value, complexity of organization, homeostasis, survival, progress, richness of experience, minimal interpersonal friction or what have you. A recent and powerful attempt by Jacques Monod looks for an ethical basis in 'the sources of science itself, in the ethic which by free choice makes knowledge the supreme value, the measure and authority of all other values'. Less ambitious and, perhaps, less precise suggestions come from Chesterton's dictum of fifty years ago that morality like a painting merely consists of 'drawing a line somewhere'. Others are based on the possibly naive notion that consideration and concern for other people should replace as *the* cardinal virtue such previously accepted supreme ones as, say, premarital chastity. Or still as another simple-minded notion one might suggest that justice toward fellow-man, rather than a commitment to any given social system, might replace the current criteria of good citizenship of paying taxes, voting, and law and order. Or the suggestion that such criteria might be based on the formulation by Sir Macfarlane Burnet who once said: 'the problem of today is how to use the intelligence of a relatively small number of men and women to devise ways by which patterns of behaviour laid down in a million years can be modified, tricked and twisted if necessary to allow a tolerable human existence in a crowded world'. Or one might refer to the biological bill of rights by Stanford University's Karl Pribram. I will not say any more than list its items: (1) Equal opportunity (liberty); (2) territory (property); (3) personal identity (integrity, reproduction, suicide); (4) humanity (happiness). Finally, I personally agree with Michael Polanyi that no chemical analysis or microscopic examination can prove that a man who bears false witness is immoral.

Are these considerations unprecedented in the history of mankind? It does not matter too much. For the majority of people in the past, standards of behaviour, of action and of social interaction, though having evolved just as other social processes and institutions, were *codified* by authority. The ethical and moral guidelines of the past have developed partly on the basis of democratic pressures, partly on the basis of service to special interests (including those of the class of priests), partly as a result of impact of individual leaders, whose motivations in turn may have been based on either, or on various rational and sometimes irrational but functional (for example as in faith healing) considerations. Guidelines have developed on still other factors too complex, too obscure, too controversial, and too dependent on individual and subjective views of religion and ethics, to discuss here. The only point that I would like to make is that all of these guidelines have had to reconcile the conflicting interests of the individual and of the group. This is to my mind a fundamental problem of human behaviour. A recent attempt was made by Raymond Cattell to resolve this conflict by asserting that it simply does not exist. I am less than sure about that. I think it is demonstrable that selection for egoistic behaviour has been more stringent than selection for altruism. In other words, biologically we may be more ego- than group-oriented. This even though, as Hobbes said, 'The life of an individual outside a group is solitary, nasty, brutish and brief'.

The decision-makers
But aside from Burnet's opinion that it will be the activities of a few people that shall bring us salvation, the question still exists as to what the decision-making process in behaviour should be. It is possible that at least modern Western society might conclude on theoretical grounds that we must rely on consensus value judgments; that is, on those arrived by some democratic process. Intuitively, I personally am sympathetic towards this solution more than to the claims of the new class of priests; be they the scientists, physicians, engineers, politicians or Pentagon thinkers. But, alas, the facts of life suggest that it makes little sense to rely on the democratic process to determine the exact speed of light, to decide on the value of *pi,* or for that matter, to select textbooks of biology for California high schools. On the other hand, delegating decisions of this sort to the modern priests can be just as unhappy. In biology, iatrocracy, the rule by physicians, can be fatal! Thomas Szasz, was, of course, right in suggesting that, as an example, abortion relates to medical judgment exactly as capital punishment relates to electrical engineering. Furthermore, quoting Dr·Kersten

Anér (this volume): '*élites* are good for a lot of things, but not for deciding what *élites* are good for'. And so we do have a dilemma. The only solution I foresee will come from courses and curricula presuming to *inform* the future arbiters of mankind's destiny.

The confrontation between individual freedom and group welfare is a central fact of existence. Another one is that doing nothing about these issues is just as full of consequences for humanity as doing something. I shall shortly give you a concrete example of this.

Often, a course of action may be deduced from the possibility of action, or, as it has been said, if a technology is available, somebody will use it, although the reality of this so-called technological imperative is under debate. Decisions that are made by whoever makes them and by whatever processes they are arrived at should be directed to some kind of good. Imprecise as Jeremy Bentham's ethic was expressed, the greatest good for the greatest number may not be terribly far wrong.

Some specific examples

Now let me give you two or three examples of specific issues that already face us. I shall not consider all of them in depth; they are merely a sampling of the wide range of problems with which we have to come to grips.

Artificial insemination

Let us examine the practice of artificial insemination with donor sperm (AID). In itself, it is not new, but the legal issues it raises are only now coming into the open. True enough the first court decision on the subject was recorded in 1883. It dealt with an unsuccessful suit by a Bordeaux physician to collect a fee for performing the service (which, parenthetically, did not result in conception). In the USA, however, the first court case did not arise until 1945. Several bills about AID have been introduced in the legislatures in various states but few had been enacted in law. In fact, the 1970 California statute which reads: 'The husband of a woman who bears a child as a result of artificial insemination shall be considered the father of that child . . . if he consented in writing to the artificial insemination' is, I believe, only the second one on the books in any of the states. An earlier one was a 1947 New York City Sanitation Department ordinance regulating the donation of semen, requiring testing it for venereal disease and Rh-blood grouping of the donor. There is also on record a resolution by the New York State Legislature limiting collection, buying and selling of semen for AID to qualified physicians. And this, mind you, in the face of the fact that in this country there are apparently upwards of 20,000 such inseminations a year!

The legal issues are numerous. Thus, in law, it is not at all clear that AID is licit. Some courts have ruled the procedure adulterous, though the California Supreme Court decision said it was not. In one of the finest examples of the legal mind at work, worthy of *The New Yorker*, the opinion reads: 'Adultery is defined as "the voluntary sexual intercourse of a married person with a person other than the offender's husband or wife". It has been suggested that the doctor and the wife commit adultery by the process of artificial insemination. Since the doctor may be a woman, or the husband himself may administer the insemination by a syringe, this is patently absurd; to consider it an act of adultery with the donor, who at the time of insemination may be a thousand miles away or may even be dead, is equally absurd.'

Nevertheless in some states the issue of whether AID is 'criminal battery' or rape has been raised, and many other legal issues are still not resolved. In some states AID children are illegitimate, in others not. This involves not only inheritance and property rights, but custody of the children in case of divorce, and responsibility for support by the legal rather than biological father, who usually is unknown. It happens that the same chapter of the California Penal Code which declares the husband who consents to the impregnation of his wife with a donor's semen is the legal father also has a section making it a misdemeanor for an adult child not to provide for an indigent parent. What parent?

The sperm donor's usual anonymity leads to still other questions which I need not enter here. Let me only ask whether eutelegenesis, that is positive eugenics or voluntary germ choice, is possible if anonymity of donors is maintained? And if not, then the Pandora's box of legal issues concerning the rights and duties of all parties is really opened.

The Green Revolution

I want to move to a completely different area where another question can be raised. This is a matter of greater social and ethical significance than my first example. You, no doubt, have all heard of the Green Revolution, the explosion of agricultural know-how in food production for the underdeveloped hungry part of the world. The improvement in yield has in part been attributed to genetics, that is to production by selective breeding of superior varieties of grains (largely wheat and rice), also to improvement in husbandry practices, to the use of fertilizers, and to pest control. I need not say much on the confrontation between farming interests and proponents of strict control of environmental pollution. The DDT debate, for instance, still rages on. I rather want to address myself to a broader ethical issue: do we in the USA really know what we, as the wealthiest country in the world, are doing in our vigorous promotion, not only of the Green Revolution, but of

Protestant-ethic humanitarianism, towards our less fortunate brethren of Asia, South America and Africa?

At first blush, according to any reasonable moral standard, we, who have so much, must help our less privileged fellow-men to achieve a longer, more comfortable, happier life, which alas, includes the means not only to conceive, but to raise large families to maturity. To do nothing but watch hunger and pestilence rampant obviously does not fit this ethic. But what are we really doing? We are helping the developing countries to increase their populations, to accelerate depletion of their resources, to strain their carrying capacity to an intolerable level, if not in the current generation, then in the future.

I do not want to enter the debate as to whether there is a real danger in population explosion, or the ever continuing argument between advocates of suasion and of coercion in limiting population growth. Nor do I need to say much on our schizophrenic position of developing population control methods and devices in the same laboratories which produce anti-sterility drugs leading to quintuplets or, God save the mark, dodecatuplets. It is a fact that while the Green Revolution is being hailed and glorified with a Nobel prize for one of its architects, that while India and the Philippines last year proclaimed themselves self-sufficient in cereal grains, this year [1973] India is in the throes of another famine and the Philippines are threatened with one. I take little comfort in the fact that this year's famine is not as severe as the last one. Hopes for technology to keep up with a population which increases by fifty million a year are wishful dreaming. To say that *something* restoring a balance between population growth and food or energy resources will turn up, is merely indulging in what Lord Morley a good many years ago labelled as a fatuous and self-deluding hope.

Whenever we provide the technology to save lives while we contribute to the exhaustion of resources and to the destruction of the environments of underdeveloped countries, essentially the price for our smug satisfaction with our good deeds today is brutality to human beings of tomorrow. What then should we do? Nothing at all? Should we try to maintain such primitive societies as the Bedouins or the nomadic tribes of Turkey at marginal levels of subsistence? Or what? Inaction, or *any* kind of conceivable action, seem to lead to equally immoral results. The worst course would be one which leads to irreversible consequences. But, alas, we do not even know enough to evaluate this possibility. There, it seems to me, is a real dilemma.

Abortion
Turning to still another level of dispute, let us consider abortion. Again,

eugenics — science of improving population by controlling breeding for desirable inherited characteristics.

the problem has been with us for a long time. But the concatenation of medical and genetical advances, with relaxation of rigid religious attitudes, has made the issue of much greater significance today. It involves ethical, biological, medical, legal and other problems. In Japan, for instance, legalized abortion became common as an instrument of social policy directed to checking population growth. Interestingly enough, it had genetic consequences not at all contemplated by the planners. Down's syndrome and Rh incompatibility were both reduced as was the opportunity for natural selection, consequent on the drop of the variance of family size.

I doubt that abortion as a birth control device would gain ready acceptance in many Western countries. But, therapeutic abortion justi-fied by the health of the mother or the health and welfare of the child, or, again, by eugenic considerations, is beginning to receive wider acceptance. The religious and ethical objections are centred on the notion that abortion is murder of the unborn child. The opposite camp questions how someone unborn could be deprived of life. Some Catholic theologians and jurists reject any kind of abortions; others draw a line based on such considerations as the mother's health. Still others are undecided as to the moment when a foetus can be considered a living being. This ranges from conception to birth. For instance, Aristotle, anticipating Talmudic law, pinpointed the first movement of the baby in the womb as the beginning of life. Curiously enough, for purposes of child support the California Penal Code considers 'a child conceived but not yet born is to be deemed an existing person'. For other pur-poses court rulings (not yet definitive) do not consider foetuses as living persons. The argument goes on. Recently, James Watson was bold enough to suggest that not only early abortion, but return to the ancient Greek practice of infanticide of grossly defective new-borns, need be considered as an instrument of socio-medical policy. And at the same time a bill severely restricting abortions is introduced in the US Senate.

An example of questions that arise when abortion laws become per-missive is provided by a small public opinion study of Oregon coeds. As you no doubt know, it is now technically possible to control the sex of one's children by amniocentesis; that is determination from cells in the amniotic fluid of the chromosome constitution of the foetus, and subsequent abortion if it proves to be of the undesired sex. The Oregon sample was overwhelmingly in favour of legalized abortion, but just as emphatic in adjudging sex predetermination as too trivial a reason to undergo abortion. Obviously, opinions differ on the matter.

In connection with amniocentesis and other tests of genotypes, a

further set of problems exists. For example, screening for serious abnormalities, such as the Tay-Sachs disease, presents an economic problem.
But it is not an issue of dollars only.

Tay-Sachs is a metabolic disease involving absence of the enzyme
component Hexosaminidase A controlled by a recessive gene, and
usually leading to a lethal outcome at approximately two to four years
of age. The frequency of the disease is relatively high only in Ashkenaz, that is Eastern European, Jews. Thus, of the expected annual
incidence of fifty-two babies born with the disease in the USA every
year, forty come from parents classified as Jewish, even though they
form only about 3 per cent of the population. Estimates based on the
cost of amniocentesis and of therapeutic abortion when needed, indicate that screening for heterozygosity of all US Jews under thirty who
marry, and abortion of the diseased genotypes, would cost about 5.7
million dollars. If no screening is done, hospitalization costs for maintaining the defective babies till death would amount to some 35 million
dollars. Screening of non-Jews would cost $78 million, while the costs
saved by eliminating the few Tay-Sachs foetuses would amount to only
10.5 million dollars. Suppose somebody would seriously propose investment for such screening and suppose that technical manpower for it
were available. Would our priorities be based on considering saving of
$30 million in the first case, and loss of $68 million in the second?
Since these computations were made, cheaper techniques for screening
carriers by assaying tears for Hexosaminidase A have been announced,
but this does not change the principle.

A somewhat different problem may exist in screening for certain
chromosomal abnormalities, for example, XYY. It has been suggested,
though the evidence is not all conclusive, that such individuals are
prone to be anti-social and populate correctional institutions in higher
than a random proportion. Whether this is true or not, would any
purpose be served in identifying XYY individuals? Is it not possible
that such identification might lead to a self-fulfilling prophecy, so that
these unfortunate carriers of chromosome aberrations would, because
of their diagnosis, become criminals?

Problems of the future
I think these various examples illustrate some of the issues raised by
modern biology. There are many others. Merely to mention a few:
priorities in organ transplants; the question as to when a potential donor
is really dead; the forensic tangles of sperm bank errors and possibility
of malpractice suits, when by error a child is sired not by the husband;
euthanasia, especially if success in prolongation of the life span beyond

the period when it can be enjoyed, if not in contemplative, then in recreational activities, is attained; and many, many others including the ultimate of brain, or as Sir John Eccles prefers, whole body transplants. If one includes psychology in our area of discussion, then the problem of differences in intelligence, and what to do about them educationally, arises. Further afield are others posed by the possibility of manipulating human behaviour by physical, chemical, or psychological means. It is clear that these concern not only scientists, physicians, legislators and theologians, but all of us. Manipulation of individual genotypes and (barely possible) genes; the prospects of cloning (to be used to replicate the genetic endowments of geniuses or to produce armies, as if from Cadmus' dragon teeth), the putting of human chromosomes into apes for research or possibly various nefarious purposes; the production of test-tube or surrogate mother babies (prenatal adoption), or multi-parental mosaics, or what not, are all parts of scenarios that have been previewed.

We are supposed, by futurologists to be on the threshold of anabiosis or cryogeny, that is, freezing human beings before death and thawing them out at the appropriate time. Thus, if there is at a given moment a surplus of, say, archbishops, they could be put into cold storage and brought back when needed. Or, somebody dying from a currently incurable disease could be frozen until the cure has been found. Think of the Roman holiday this would produce for lawyers settling property inheritance and the like!

All of these may not be overly extravagant prospects, since we already have our hands full with immediate urgent questions that are as difficult. The fundamental one is how to anticipate the potentially problem-generating areas. One school of thought suggests that we can escape these problems by a moratorium on research. It is hard for me to believe that there can be too much knowledge. Yet, establishing priorities for research, the regulation of technologies which can bring mankind to grief and, above all, of workable metaethical principles seem to me to have the first call. And once more we face the closely related twin dilemmas: what or who are to be the source of the ethical guidelines, and who is to make decisions with the infinite regressed corollary as to who guards the guardians?

These problems are especially poignant if one goes along with the idea that man has arrived at a watershed in human history, at the cosmic threshold of not only understanding his origin, but of acquiring the capacity for designing his biological future. Many of those who think that actual tinkering with the DNA of single human genes is an unattainable dream still believe this. But there are also dissenting voices.

One of the greatest minds of our times, J. B. S. Haldane, in the year of his death, less than ten years ago, raised severe doubts about the view that we already can, should we choose to do so, control our future evolution. Aside from the fact that the practice of gene therapy is still a dream, Haldane posed the thought that there is not even one gene now found in the majority of our species which we would wish to become more common, if not universal. (He may be wrong in this: I imagine that the normal allele of the Tay-Sachs gene falls into this category.) Furthermore, he maintained, we do not know how much heterozygosity and at what loci we desire change. Nor do we know what the environment of our descendants will be like, and hence are unable to tell the direction towards which our manipulation of the human gene pool should take. Should it be increased resistance to gamma radiation, or properties which would make men successful planetary colonists, or special psychological equipment to live in a crowded and polluted world? Or what? Haldane asks how many Shakespeares, Marxes or Gandhis we should have in an optimal situation, and concludes by saying: 'I am glad to think that we do not know enough genetics even to misdirect our evolution seriously, much less to direct it'.

Yet many others do not find his doubts convincing. Personally, I find the claims for early availability of technical means, for genetic or educational engineering practices to enable us to direct human evolution, more plausible than the assertion that we really do have enduring social goals and scales of good and bad at hand. There are any number of instances of values changing within a single generation, and they are not the only ones that are generated by opposite goals pursued by different contemporary human societies. The great geneticist, H. J. Muller, one of the most vigorous proponents of eutelegenesis on humanist grounds, has moved, in the course of his lifetime, from Marx, Lenin and Sun Yat Sen as the most admirable types of potential sperm donors, to Darwin, Einstein and Schweitzer, simply because he found Stalin's practices different from Stalin's avowed ideals. Such arbitrariness in itself, when summed over the aims of a given society, may even produce an anti-evolutionary or braking effect, in the sense that it might favor maintenance of current attitudes and forms of existence over changes.

In fact, one conclusion that seems valid is that if man were fully in control over differential reproduction within his species, he would more likely attempt to conserve his dominant position on earth than to permit a superior (even according to his own standards) form to replace him. It works not only at the social but also at the biological level. Suppose (to borrow a concept from Haldane) mutations for wings and for high moral character arose in man. Would the powers, whether vested in the *élite* or in the *demos,* encourage their propagation so that angels could inherit the earth? No. The seeing man in the kingdom of the blind, as H. G. Wells has so penetratingly described, is more likely to find himself with his eyes put out, than with dozens of children! It seems problematic that, in absence of a cataclysm, the currently dominant species on earth will permit itself to be replaced.

Despite the fact that many of us decry conformity and speak with high favour of human diversity, I am not sure that humanity would actively promote the disappearance of *Homo sapiens* in favour of *Homo superior.*

Portents and promises

I have already covered some of the biological or genetic factors. Hence, I want to move on to a listing of portents and promises largely of environmental and psychological significance. But, it is important to remember and to emphasize that there is a mutual feedback between nature and nurture. A thermo-nuclear holocaust will have a biological effect in producing deleterious mutations or in changing, at least temporarily, sex ratios.

Emergence of a dictatorship can lead to imposition of sterilization or detention programs for certain classes of the population, for example, those adjudged to be aberrant or insane by virtue of either their *descent* or *dissent*. And changes in mankind's gene pool are bound to have social sequelae. It is then only too obvious that the type of evolution that man is currently undergoing is increasingly less organic, and more and more, as various people have called it, exosomatic, exogenetic or psychosocial.

My emphasis on the negative potentialities is possibly due to the fact that we live in an intellectually analytic age, characterized by breakdown of the whole into its elements. This is witnessed among other things by the trends in the art, music and literature of this century. The re-synthesis of the identifiable elements into a new integrated entity or body of beliefs and attitudes is yet to come in various areas of human endeavour. And if this view is conceded, the difficulties can be seen much clearer than the opportunities, and the negative trends appear more conspicuous than the hopeful signs. In brief then, the threats:

Nuclear or chemical and biological warfare

In the ultimate, this hazard may lead to total extinction of mankind. But even a limited unleasing of atomic weapons would have not only

immediate repercussions in terms of loss of life and increases in mutation rate, but also probably far-reaching effects on ethical standards
in international behaviour. I am sure that there are some who support
the position that a partial nuclear catharsis might expose once and for
all the folly of war. This is not a defensible view. Historically, we still
continue waging war after war to end war.

Ascendancy of the military and managerial classes

More generally this is the *obsolescence of town-hall democracy* (even
in a representative guise), underlying many of the forms of government in the Western world. In a way, this threat is the result of continued technological progress. While the accelerating increases in mastery
over environment, and the medical advances in controlling disease and
prolonging life represent proud achievements of modern man, they
also create problems in administering and decision making. In many
countries, we witness the rise of dictatorship in varying degrees by the
military, by the industrial establishment, by plutocratic elements, or by
political parties. It hardly seems likely that any group in power will
relinquish its control voluntarily. Yet, should such control be wrested
from them by democratic forces, history tells us that usually the successful rebels merely impose the rule by their own *élite*.

Environmental pollution, population growth, and depletion of resources

The conflict between conservation and our living standards, con-
veniences and luxuries is obvious. Will the general mass of people be
willing to adopt the simple life and give up their material comforts for
posterity? Yet, who controls the right to propagate?

Breakdown of the social fabric and of moral standards

This unhappy situation is really at the back of our present ethical
dilemmas. The morality of medieval ages, of Puritan England, or of
Prohibition United States is not necessarily suited for the year 2000,
but it is a defensible position that *a* morality is needed for society to
survive. Of course, there have always been prophets, no doubt, preceding St. Cyprian and even those of the Old Testament, who were
preaching the coming end of the world and were usually derided. The
fact is, however, that sooner or later, as one civilization replaced
another, their prophecies have been fulfilled. It may be arguable that
each successive one was an improvement over the previous one, but
it is also clear that at least short-term disasters for mankind punctuated
their progression. All of our current institutions, even as sacrosanct as
the church, the family, wholesome motherhood, or even milk drinking
are not immutable biological or social attributes. Changes in them have

occurred in the past and must occur in the future. But the problem *still* is that no comprehensive ethic for the twenty-first century has yet evolved to replace the crumbling one we have lived by, at least in theory, in our immediate past.

The rise of anti-intellectualism and of cults of unreason

This threat, alas, is apparent not only in the socialist countries, where, for example, Lysenkoism (the decimation of genetics as a discipline) and bans on free artistic and literary expression, have occurred. It was also present under fascism, when political, cultural, and personal repression of various sorts formed part of a national philosophy imposed from above. It is manifest in our own advanced society not only as a grass-root movement, but also promoted by any number of free-wheeling university instructors despite the fact that they are by definition intellectuals. Courses in witchcraft, curricula specifically barring any reference to science, technology or mathematics, all more or less essential for even semi-educated people of this generation, are evidences of this trend.

Control of the mind

The developing techniques of manipulating the human brain, and in consequence human behaviour, by hormones, drugs, and electrical stimulation most certainly present dangers if unscrupulously used. The coming of age of behavioural sciences by the beginning of the next century may be welcome because it will extend our knowledge about the most fundamental properties of man as a social animal. But just as the age of physics culminated in thermonuclear weapons, and the age of biology is posing major and unsolved problems, so do behaviour sciences have a potential for conflict between the good from scientific advances and their possible abuse. I need only to give you two quotes from José Delgado who is in the forefront of research in this area: (1) 'The question rather than "What is man?" should be "What kind of man are we going to construct?" ' and (2) 'The inviolability of the brain is only a social construct like nudity.' No comments.

Racial strife

The explosiveness of this factor in a repressive white controlled society such as South Africa, and the anti-Asian movement in Uganda, or others closer to home, does not call for documentation. Here is a single biological example of a relatively trivial kind, of the relationship between cultural and organic evolution: some ten or fifteen years ago prognoses and time estimates for the emergence of an eventual single human gene pool in the USA could be made on the assumption of random mating between blacks and whites. The anticipated breakdown in assortative mating by colour presumably would result in a neo-North American race with a distribution of skin colours ranging around a mean just slightly darker in skin colour than the present day whites. But the subsequent rise of the black movement in search of an identity, and of ideas of biological segregation advocated by its militant members, currently suggests that we may wind up in two non-overlapping (so far as pigmentation goes) sub-populations as the end-product. But, obviously the trend may be reversed again in the next ten years.

Now to turn briefly to some hopeful signs: the first one is *increase of control over environment, including elimination of disease, conquest of physical suffering and, perhaps, of death.* All of these raise as many problems as they solve, especially since the uses to which knowledge is put can be positive or negative, depending upon one's outlook on any specific applications of it, and upon the motivations of those in control of these applications. The second: *rise in education and standards of living.* Whatever the pitfalls we face are, the possibilities of avoiding them can only be enhanced by spread of information, by rational behaviour and by elimination of want (development of these may in part depend on psychological engineering, for example in changing food acceptance and other attitudes). A computer and robot civilization need not be based on a completely materialistic outlook. It is not an obligatory consequence of the direction of our cultural evolution that mankind will transform itself into a pleasure-oriented society in which leisure will be devoted to programmed dreaming or, what has been called, wholesome degeneracy. We should be able to do better. The furthering of esthetic ideals, of possibilities of self-actualization, of fulfilment of man's potential for expressing himself both as an individual and as a member of a group, the development of loyalties to increasingly more inclusive entities from self, to family, to parish, to country, to the world at large—all are attainable with the conquest over hunger, disease, toil, hatred and war, which technology can make possible.

The third and most encouraging sign is the *persistence of man's hope in the face of threats to his ideals.* Of the many human traits, arising as a result of organic and cultural evolution, the most 'human' ones are those dealing with psychological attitudes and behaviour patterns. They include extension of capacities to communicate across space and time, powers of abstraction, imagination and 'displacement' (that is, the ability of thinking or speaking of things in the past or future or of things imagined), inventiveness, the sense of beauty and of the sacred, the realization of personal mortality at least for the nonce, the high degree of educability, and the possibility of single individuals of outstanding mentality to leave an everlasting impact on human existence. All of these can be harnessed for the good of our own species without undue sacrifice of material values. These properties and others like them, have, indeed, produced an altruism of a higher order than that seen anthropomorphically in patterns of behaviour of soldier or worker insects. In its superior manifestation this altruism concerns the welfare of descendants as yet unborn. And this altruism, whatever its origin, may well counteract most of the threats that I have listed.

Let me then finish by a paraphrase of the concluding sentence of a book of mine with which a few of you may be familiar. The ethics of the decision-making in the contemporary world are not clear, but the development of an effective and just machinery for this process as it concerns individuals and society should have a high place on mankind's agenda. Only an informed society can accomplish this task. That is why understanding of genetics, of population biology and of the evolutionary outlook is an indispensable ingredient in the cultural baggage of every educated person.

CHAPTER 3

Ethical issues raised by eugenics:
an orthodox and Asian perspective

Paul Verghese

Syrian Orthodox Theological Seminary, Kerala, India

Do we all take it for granted that we know what we mean when we say 'ethical issues raised by eugenics'? For me it is not so clear. Is the assumption that in every situation there is a given choice between two actions, one of which is 'right' and the other 'wrong'? Is it also assumed that we can prescribe for others such 'right' actions and proscribe certain 'wrong' ones? Also that we can describe in words all that belongs to a situation, including its components, its possibilities and the options it offers us? I cannot personally make any of these assumptions.

All that can be hoped for in such discussions is illumination, not settlement, of the situations confronting man as he gains more power over the genes which are so decisive for the life of man and all living beings.

Illumination is required for three different types of situations. One is that of the professional who has to exercise the power of interfering with the life of another person. The other is that of the pastor who has to give counsel to people who have to make decisions about themselves or their loved ones. The third is that of the legislator who makes laws which are binding on all people. Ethical discussion has to take account of all three types of decisions.

The question of the norm

The assumption in most ethical discussion is that there are certain given norms on the basis of which we can make ethical decisions. But reflection reveals the fragility of these so-called norms. We have not yet proceeded in human reflection to the point where we can verbally capture the meaning of the word 'good'. And so long as that is true, all articulated norms for ethical conduct will remain essentially frail and fragile. We find it difficult to accept the fact, and in stubborn hope continue the pursuit of ethical norms.

In Asian society, the individual ethical consciousness has not been developed to the same extent as in the West. The Asian often makes his decisions on the basis of social traditions of long standing antiquity or on the grounds of pure expediency. The question of abortion, for example, would bring out the nature of this Asian ambivalence. In many countries in Asia daughters are still under the protection of their parents till the time of marriage, irrespective of age. If an unmarried daughter gets pregnant, the parents will be so shocked in some cases as to disown the daughter altogether. That is the social tradition. Middle class families would not normally resort to abortion because it is against the social tradition. But nowadays a new culture whose values are basically pragmatic is being superimposed on the old culture where social tradition played a decisive and normative role. Today, therefore, parents belonging to any class may resort to abortion in the case of a pregnant unmarried daughter, especially if it can be achieved without much risk, pain or publicity, even if it costs some money. Social stigma is even more feared than death. People in Asia in general do not make their ethical decisions after systematic and agonising moral reflection on the options available, based on given precise norms. We oscillate between social tradition and immediate expediency, and therefore reflection on the basis of ethical norms plays a much less powerful role in Asian society than in the West.

The three existential perspectives

Take amniocentesis and selective abortion, to see how a typical Asian family would react to the issues. Normally mothers do not go to a doctor in mid-pregnancy unless there is something abnormal. But if she does, then the medical doctor's authority is so great that he can do any kind of examination including cytogenetic and biochemical analysis of the amniotic fluid. If the doctor pronounces the foetus to be genetically defective, most parents' reactions would be governed by the confidence they have in the doctor and in the hospital where the examination was made. They may, if they can afford it, want to consult another physician in whom they have more confidence. But if they are convinced that the infant is going to be significantly and *visibly* defective as to be liable to be socially unacceptable, then most Asian parents would consent to abortion. It is an intuitive reaction, not a reflected decision on the basis of norms and principles.

But that is from the parents' point of view. If we now look at the same problem from the physician's point of view we will see that he has to take into account a number of factors: possible damage to the foetus through insertion of the needle into the amniotic sac; the limited reliability of any tests of this kind; and finally, since useful amniocentesis usually takes place after at least three months of pregnancy, abortion at this advanced stage may involve the risk of physical and emotional damage to the mother.

From the third, that is the legislator's point of view, one will have to have precise specfication of the kind of degree of genetic defect that will justify abortion. Not just any genetic defect will be sufficient ground for seeking abortion. A very large number of genetic defects can be coped with by our modern medical facilities, and to cite Dr Bentley Glass (this symposium), myopia and allergy or gout are not adequate as genetic defects to warrant abortion. Negative eugenics does demand a parameter for measuring genetic defect, so that beyond a certain degree, it would warrant abortion. Such a norm is difficult for a society to argee upon, and is not given in absolute form in the Christian traditions. In a country like India, where the sway of professional or ethical standards is often low, due to the economic and political circumstances, legally to authorize abortion on the basis of amniocentesis would, in effect, mean legalizing abortion in any case where the physician can *certify* genetic defect. And physicians in India do certify all sorts of things, regardless of whether they are true or not.

Ethical questions in eugenics

What we have so far done is to examine the problem of an advanced pregnancy where cytogenetic and biochemical analysis has revealed major genetic defect in the foetus, from three existential perspectives, where the decisions are made on the basis of pragmatic considerations rather than theoretical principles.

Though it is not very much in the Asian temperament to make individual ethical decisions based on theoretical principles, it will be useful for me as an Asian to reveal to you some of my own theoretical perplexities, in the hope of finding illumination from minds more used to theoretical reflection.

I do not want to discuss the ethical justification for abortion here, though my perplexity in seeking to follow the debate· can only be described as enormous. I wish to limit the ethical reflection to the question of negative eugenics and positive eugenics.

In the field of negative eugenics, there are three theoretical questions which have an ethical bearing:

The question of priority

Charles Birch has raised this issue in his paper in this volume. The energy, intelligence and resources devoted to remedying genetic defects in a few individuals could be more fruitfully deployed today, to ameliorate the environment in which millions have to live everywhere in the world, in the rich countries as well as in the poor. More human beings suffer today because of the environment (physical, social, economic, cultural, political) into which they are born rather than because of the genetic equipment with which they have arrived in that environment. Theoretically therefore, while it is not a question of either/or, the priority in terms of urgency and deployment of resources has to be given to the environment problem in all its aspects, over the demands to correct the genetic equipment of a few individuals. The latter can receive only less attention and resources than the former.

The question of justice

If you take the cost factor into account as an ethical problem, it is clear that the economically poor nations of the world cannot at present undertake a nation-wide programme for compulsory amniocentesis for all pregnant women. This means amniocentesis, in the poorer countries, would remain another privilege, available to the elite and not available to the under-privileged. This constitutes a moral problem in itself.

Problems in the field of positive eugenics are related to the ones raised above in negative eugenics, but could be differently formulated:

Who decides?

The line of demarcation between the realm of life in which individuals are given the freedom to make personal decisions and that other realm where the decisions are made by society, is a shifting and often unclear one. Is there a fundamental human right called 'the right of progeny'? If I am mentally or physically defective, do I thereby lose the right to have children, to prolong the family succession or do I have to sacrifice the identity of my particular line of human succession by opting for sterilization? Should I leave it to society to decide whether I come up to the standards of what they regard to be minimal for the future of humanity, thereby accepting their probable condemnation of my genetic line, and therefore judge my particular line of human specificity and distinctiveness as unfit to survive? How does such an abdication of personal responsibility to society reflect upon our present ideas about the worth of each human person? Or are we to say some people are sufficiently worthy only to live on till death, but not worthy to have progeny?

On what basis do they decide?

What are the criteria for measuring the kind of degree of genetic defect that would warrant pre-natal abortion? To what extent are we justified as a society to deny existence to an individual likely to develop cystic fibrosis or sickle cell anaemia? In whose interest is the decision made that such individuals have no right to be born?

On what basis again would we say that cystic fibrosis or sickle cell anaemia do not warrant resort to abortion, but Down's syndrome (mongolism) does so warrant? Can we do this on the basis of the cost factor for institutionalizing a child suffering from it? Can we set down the value of a human life in terms of how much it costs to maintain it?

If we have to make such decisions either as a society or as individuals we need more clearly articulated criteria or parameters for measuring human worth. What do we in fact mean when we say 'This particular genetic strain is worth promoting; that particular strain not so'? Are we going to create a new class structure and a new scale of values, based on the parameter which we are going to use? Do we need a new elitism of those elected to continue their progeny as over, against those not so chosen?

Even if we say that such an elitism is desirable for the sake of the future of man, the practical problems connected with such a standard are enormously difficult. Are good health, an exceptional intellectual ability, great stamina and aptitude for social service the categories we are going to choose? Are all these categories genetically determined? Is all human greatness genetically conditioned? Is a society composed only of exceptionally healthy, exceptionally gifted, and exceptionally social-minded individuals subject to further and deeper corruptions springing out of the radical evil present in humanity? Do we need an ocean of mediocrity in order to foster islands of exceptional merit? Is all human suffering evil? Does not greatness often come out of suffering and deprivation rather than out of a perfect setting provided for the human being?

These and many other such questions must continue to pester us. We can ill afford to say that we will face them when they come up.

CHAPTER 4

Judging the social values of scientific advances

R. G. Edwards

Physiological Laboratory, Cambridge University, UK

A feature of our modern society is the constant succession of new moral and ethical issues arising in a changing world. Many of these issues stem from alterations in social values and attitudes towards earlier problems, and several such examples can be quoted from recent memory: permissiveness in society, the legalization of abortion, the abolition of capital punishment, the widespread abuse of drugs. A significant number also arise from medical and technical advances in specific areas of research, which challenge established ideas or open new possibilities of choice. These advances are reported regularly, often in large headlines. While the excessive publicity lavished on these advances is to be deplored, the attention they attract should be welcomed by those concerned in discussing and establishing ethical and social standards or social awareness, for the resulting discussions often concern people in widely differing professions or with widely diverging views. There appears to be no current limit to the number of these issues as science interferes more and more intimately with human affairs. Debates on the details of a particular clinical or social situation thus provide a major impetus to establishing new standards, and the manner in which such issues arise and are handled in contemporary society forms the major part of my theme.

Many of the discussions at this consultation are concerned with the prenatal detection of inherited defects in foetuses, and with genetic aspects of population. The development of prenatal diagnosis illustrates how new social situations arise from unrelated scientific or clinical discoveries, for the possibility of screening foetuses by amniocentesis arose, I believe, from observations that amniotic fluid tapped during pregnancy could be used to measure the well-being of the foetus. The concept of typing foetuses for inherited conditions arose later, and has led to debates on the ethics of practising 'eugenic' abortions, the place in society of people carrying genetic defects, and the rights of foetuses.

Many opportunities arise from such innocuous beginnings and result in the sudden emergence of social problems. Society is often unprepared for making decisions on new developments, hence a successive series of haphazard responses usually precedes the elaboration of a balanced set of judgments.

Fertilization of human ova *in vitro*

A worthwhile model, which could be of importance in genetic diagnosis and is relevant to the discussions at this symposium concerns the development of studies on the fertilization *in vitro* of human ova. The initial step was a scientific discovery far removed from any clinical work, and partly gained from animal experiments, that oocytes collected from discarded ovaries could be persuaded to 'ripen' in culture. An immediate consequence was the development of studies on the origin of certain forms of inherited human defects, such as Down's syndrome (mongolism), and on the processes of human ovulation. From this beginning arose the possibility of bringing human ovulation, fertilization and early development under a degree of control, and so provide a source of human embryos for clinical use. The primary value here lay in curing infertility by reimplanting embryos in the mother's uterus, for many thousands of couples cannot conceive because an occluded oviduct in the wife prevents spermatozoa reaching the egg and the egg from entering the uterus. Other patients could also benefit, for example, infertile men with few spermatozoa. Further clinical developments were also possible, including the identification of embryos with genetic defects even before they were implanted in the uterus, so averting the need for eugenic abortions in mid-pregnancy.

Although the advantages of such studies were clear enough, the initial response of many people was hardly enthusiastic with the realization that human eggs had to be fertilized *in vitro* in order to achieve these targets. This notion was foreign and unexpected, even to many scientists working on similar studies with animals. Part of the adverse response arose through the challenge to established social orders; previously, human conception had been intimate and personal, and the private affair of a couple, whereas it could now occur in the placid confines of a culture dish. Other responses were, predictably, based on stances long adopted on related issues. The initial response, for example of the hierarchy of the Roman Catholic Church was to declare this kind of work immoral and illicit, irrespective of its considerable potential to help with many human problems; this attitude obviously stems from the stance of this church to contraception and abortion. The scene

was confused further by the entry of a professional group of fore-
casters, including scientists, predicting the direst of consequences in
genetic engineering, notably cloning, test-tube babies and the destruction of family life, 'host' mothers and so on. Even the reimplantation
of embryos into their own mothers as a cure of infertility was considered to be non-therapeutic, because it would not cure the original
clinical condition of the patients. What a story to tell to the infertile!
Some of the arguments were offered in religious terms, such as the
assertion that human procreation is divine and unchangeable, or that
the application of a treatment to foetuses is unethical because they
cannot consent beforehand. There are many people in the world today
who must be grateful that somebody *did* interfere in conception or
foetal development without first getting the consent of the foetus, for
example in Rhesus disease. Similar objections are raised in different
clinical contexts, such as prenatal screening, where initial adverse
responses are based on accepted values and the *status quo,* even though
the new opportunities offer a choice in courses of action.

The public debate

With time, a more balanced view prevails. The issues become clear,
the benefits are seen for their true value, and the problems associated
with novel approaches recognized. Relevant opinion can come from
diverse sources for, with wider education and communication, many
people are able to evaluate opportunities of new biomedical advances.
Nevertheless, in the early phases of research and development, no-one
is capable of clarification except those directly involved in the work,
hence scientists and doctors have to undertake many of the steps necessary to publicise and explain their work, often under adverse circumstances. The lack of a press officer in many universities or institutions
provides an example of unpreparedness for the careful transmission of
information to a wide public. The initial response is thus dealt with
by scientists or doctors coping with all the issues—good and bad—
raised by others in relation to their work, and inevitably distrust of
science is raised in the public mind. Even though misunderstanding
arises in this way, it is difficult to decide who else should give a lead
to public debate. Some, but by no means all of the more irrational
responses to new developments can be attributed to the mass media,
although many others make their own contribution to the confusion.
There are some, fortunately few, professional 'ethicists' who are prepared to open public debate, although their opinions may merely reflect
their own prejudices. This weakness in the transfer of information needs

to be remedied: perhaps organizations composed of a diversity of professional men should be established to clarify and publicise new issues as they arise.

Control of research?

The successive challenges to established values arising from clinical and scientific work has resulted in a widespread feeling that research must be controlled from outside its own confines in some manner. There is a current belief that barriers must be imposed on the development of research, which will ensure that the scientist toes the line drawn by more responsible members of society, and does not become involved in developing germ warfare, nuclear weapons, and other horrors, real or imagined. Scientists are suspected of 'playing at God', unthinkingly and without cause, so that their peers must evaluate the likely effects of specific research projects more realistically than they do themselves. Another image detracts from the public idea of the scientist, for he is widely imagined to be too concerned and absorbed with his own work to appreciate the wider issues frequently raised by it. There could well be a grain of truth in this belief, and some scientists might shrink from public defence of their work, a point developed later in this article.

Can external controls be imposed on scientific research without losing more than is gained? I believe that the application of rigid external controls in 'pure' research would be an error, although more encouragement and recognition to applied research should be given than is usual in the traditional British approach. There are several reasons for adopting this attitude. The social value of most research projects cannot be classified as wholly good or bad, for the consequences of most work cannot be predicted, even by those closest to it. Pure research must be judged primarily on its immediate scientific value, and the people most capable of judging are those involved in the work itself; the meaningful imposition of objectives, and direction by outsiders, is virtually impossible. External controls would probably limit progress, for scientific research flourishes best when there are minimal restrictions on investigators. In some circumstances, for example when research involves patients, the nature of the work is carefully watched, but this stipulation does not change the need to avoid interference wherever possible. The ethical problems arise as 'pure' research is put into practice or its development has taken place with this intention in mind. But the responsibility for putting theoretical ideas and concepts into practice is not an issue concerning most research scientists, nor is it likely to be their sole responsibility should the occasion arise in their work. These reasons lead me to reject the notion of peer controls over most scientific research, although there is no doubt that a considerable degree of control can be imposed on particular types of research if by no other means than deliberate limitation of research funds. Should certain forms of research be curtailed in this way, for reasons concerned with vague values and concepts, then some potential beneficiaries of the application of the work will be deprived of clinical support through the failure to develop projects as quickly as possible.

The opposition to this plea for the freedom of the scientist can be predicted. Attitudes will be expressed that scientists are developing techniques of considerable power detrimental to mankind, merely in pursuit of their own ego and satisfaction, and proposals offered that society must impose value judgments concerned not with the research itself but with potential consequences of it. I believe that such controls should be exerted at the point of application of research, for such judgements will involve a complex set of values including national priorities, patient care, cost/benefit and other broad values, including the ethical issues. This is the actual situation found in most hospitals concerned with research, where committees are appointed to oversee new developments involving research treatments on patients. In stressing the importance of the applied scientist in issues affecting social standards, I am not suggesting that the 'pure' scientist should refrain from commenting on the potential application of his work, or from complaining loud and long if he disagrees with its applied development, for the contributions to social debates by highly articulate and trained people is obviously one of the safeguards against misapplication.

Ethical decisions

The wider problems associated with scientific and clinical research thus arise when decisions are being taken to apply new concepts in practice. There is no ethical judgement in knowing that amniocentesis is possible: difficulties arise when decisions are being made to use it with the intention of detecting and aborting foetuses with various defects. Judgments on the application of such research are likely to be made by people in various professions; the scientist and doctor will have a part in decision making, for they appreciate the technical issues, are in close touch with patients, and must put new ideas into practice, but their role is limited. The decisions to be made will involve administrators and lawyers: they will necessitate the spending of large sums of money on a national scale, or the choosing of the kind of patient most likely to benefit from particular advances. Decision-making will thus involve more and more people when the application becomes imminent, and various factors—financial, legal, ethical—may determine the introduction of new ideas into established practice.

Yet scientists and doctors engaged in new work must not underrate their authority on contributing to these judgements, especially since they will be in the forefront of new scientific and medical advances. The issues to be decided are neither negligible nor declining in importance to mankind, for they concern the fundamental idea of life, death and the quality of life. By knowingly discussing issues and initiating action, these professional men can provide standards of debate and behaviour for the rest of society to accept or reject. An intriguing aspect of the ensuing debates is that some of the fundamental points previously debated in more abstract forms are brought into sharper focus, for example, the beginning of life or the time of death, and so an immediacy and relevancy is imparted to earlier philosophical or theoretical discussions. There is obviously a need for interdisciplinary discussions of new issues, and fortunately there has been no shortage of symposia on the ethical and moral issues during recent years. While many of these debates have included re-statements of set positions, others have shown the value of a comprehensive approach by revealing the limitations of each profession taking their own separate decisions. There are also other constraints on doctors engaged in applying new clinical studies, some being exerted through professional organisations and others through the local environment. Inevitably, a wide number of people are drawn into such work, for example, other doctors, nurses and patients, so that debate can often begin at the local level.

Much of the initiative in stimulating discussion must arise from within the scientific and medical professions and should include the open publication and discussion of results as they are obtained. Once debate has begun, it can spread widely through the media of mass communication, often resulting in a distortion of the true issues. The doctor or scientist can thus be thrust into roles previously allotted to more public figures, such as politicians, theologians and others involved in creating standards or framing courses of action, a situation that can be expensive in terms of time, effort and reputation. Such a role may not be accepted by some scientists and doctors in the front line of public enquiry who prefer to shun public discussion of their work, and who are anyway insufficiently trained in judging social issues or even in communicating with non-scientists. But it is as unrealistic for them to claim that they proceed with their work unhindered, as to suggest that outside people should control what they do. There must be an ongoing debate between the professional men and the wider public, and the difficult issues have to be debated widely and explained by the press and other media of communication. The development of many organizations to debate and publicise social responsibility in science illustrated this need, and shows that this position is now accepted by at least some members of the scientific and medical community.

Discussions on the social consequences of research with people from diverse backgrounds can sometimes be more stimulating than carrying out the original research work itself. Such involvement in public debate need not be a burden to be shouldered unwillingly or reluctantly, for scientists and doctors are by no means the sole fount of wisdom, even on their own affairs! There are safeguards in such wide communication, for many challenges will arise not only from within the scientific and medical professions, but also from sources outside these specialities, including political pressure. The careers of those involved in early years of family planning provide a commentary on public pressures that can be brought to bear. Mistaken concepts in genetics led to suggestions—even heard today—that the 'unfit' or criminal should be sterilized in order to reduce the frequency of undesirable genes in the population, yet genetic analyses have shown such measures to be ineffective eugenically. Such examples provide salutory evidence of the power of new developments to provoke reactions at all levels of society. Situations such as eugenic abortion or AID thus call for the widest debate, since emotions are easily stirred when the rights and prejudices of different people are in conflict.

The existing public debate concerning the fertilization of human eggs *in vitro* illustrates many of the comments made above. Some of the viewpoints expressed have been too narrow and restricted by personal fears in a particular professional field, rather than a commentary on the wider issues involved. The judgments of some scientists for example, have been mesmerized by impractical concepts of genetic engineering, or by misunderstanding of the population problem in relation to medical advances, for no doctor could be justified in withholding urgent treatment through fears of cloning or because of the excessive fecundity of the population at large. Some theologians were tempted to push their concepts on the sanctity of life *in utero* to such an extreme that their judgement of contemporary clinical developments became meaningless. The new methods often offer a choice—perhaps a very difficult choice—demanding a reappraisal of attitudes based on earlier knowledge and ability. Nor have such criticisms stood the test of time as judged by comments at various symposia, for such stances were irrelevant to the clinical values and problems raised by the work and often obscured debate on genuine difficulties raised by it.

Even now, several of the real issues involved in fertilization *in vitro* have not been fully analysed, and I will take one example to illustrate this point: some laboratories are prepared to develop programmes on fertilization *in vitro* and early growth of the embryo as a scientific study, thus accepting the view that human embryos can be deliberately initiated in the laboratory and then destroyed later. This situation is very different from that occurring in clinical studies where the embryos are used in attempts to cure infertility, and it cannot be justified by reference to current social practices where embryos or foetuses conceived accidentally are aborted, for example the use of IUD or menstrual aspiration for birth control. Accepting fertilization *in vitro* as a laboratory study in its own right can thus lead to the establishment of values about early human growth, including the assumption that these stages of life are expendable for scientific purposes. This assumption is also made in other kinds of experimental work including the testing of new contraceptive agents, where foetuses resulting from 'failures' are later aborted. There is obviously some justification for such work, for the social benefits could be considerable; nevertheless, those foetuses aborted during the trials were not conceived with much hope of their onward growth to full term. In contrast, clinical work aimed at embryo transfer includes at least an attempt to preserve the life of the embryo and nurture it to full term, and the intention of the work is to establish life and avert the origin of birth defects. Obviously, more attention must be given to the nature of foetal rights and to the role of the experimenter in such kinds of work.

Another group of experiments must also be examined closely, namely where an aborted mid-trimester foetus is kept alive as long as possible—usually a few hours—and used in experimental studies during this time. One justification of this type of work is that the foetus would die anyway, but this attitude begs some questions, such as whether it feels any pain as the experimental work is performed.

A sense of realism must be maintained in judging the social value of new scientific and clinical advances. Many doctors have to make ethical decisions in the day-to-day course of their work. Changes in public attitudes can occur very quickly as new opportunities are understood, leaving the professionals in the rearguard of change. On occasions, patients have decided certain issues while doctors were still debating them: women with infertile husbands, or those at risk from the birth of a child with inherited defects, have conceived extramaritally while the doctors were still debating the acceptability of AID. Taking an ethical stance implies that its consequences must be accepted, hence those who condemn AID or eugenic abortions must clarify the value of their alternatives to those patients and doctors faced with the application of such methods. I find great difficulty in accepting the notion that conception is divine as a reason or solace for withholding help from infertile couples yearning for their own children, or that the sacredness of life is sufficient reason to avoid aborting all foetuses with severe genetic defects. A relevant point in this connection has been made many times over; if God gave us our intelligence and ability, we were presumably meant to use them. A 'head in sand' policy of adhering to preconceived notions in the face of new ideas and approaches is a short cut to irrelevancy.

Perhaps past experience will serve us well in framing a rational attitude to further advances, for there is certainly a greater awareness now of the possibilities and limitations of science and medicine. New ethical issues are bound to arise in fields such as the control of behaviour, the inheritance of intelligence and other complex human characteristics, and these will also require further adaptations by society. There is no doubt that society can adapt to such challenges, and that the quality of life can be greatly improved by their judicious application. Let us hope that conferences such as the present one will help to ensure that the problems raised by them are discussed freely and sensibly.

CHAPTER 5

Ethical problems raised by genetics

Bentley Glass

State University of New York at Stony Brook, USA

'Genetic engineering' or 'genetic manipulation', terms frequently used in discussions of the future implications of genetic discoveries, really mean little or nothing distinct from the older term 'eugenics'. Inasmuch as they are highly perjorative terms, implying that strong measures of some kind are to be imposed upon a population without personal consent, I believe they should be avoided. It is important to recognize that geneticists already engineer the genomes of whatever plants and animals they wish, especially the domestic animals and cultivated plants, by applying conventional methods of breeding and selection. All the triumphs of applied genetics have been achieved in that way. It is therefore crucial to consider whether the anticipated new methods about to be discovered and applied to mankind are either more effective in modifying a population than the conventional ones, or are more likely to be seized as instruments of tyrannical authority. We must recognize that at present, in spite of the abundant evidence that conventional methods could be used to breed desired types of humans, no such programme exists anywhere. Those that have been tried, on occasion, proved ineffectual and were abandoned (Glass 1972a).

Inasmuch as many critics of eugenics have raised objections to the imposition of restraints upon the supposed paramount right of individuals to breed as they desire, let it be stated emphatically that virtually all human societies have imposed regulations upon the freedom of marriage and procreation. Most human societies have banned incest by law or taboo, in spite of the fact that royal families have not infrequently attempted to perpetuate their characteristics and to hold their sacred power by close inbreeding—even brother-sister mating. Many societies have practised infanticide whenever a newborn child was manifestly deformed. More commonly, social ostracism and seclusion in a penal or mental institution has been visited upon persons who were adjudged criminal or insane, or who had loathsome diseases such as leprosy. Compulsory sterilization was inflicted upon selected individuals, in order to produce eunuchs for house slaves, or *castrati* for singers. Into very recent times, many states of the USA practised compulsory sterilization of mental defectives; but the laws whereby this was enforced have since the 1930's fallen into disfavour and are now little used, although often remaining on the books.

Such measures as those just described, although possibly of surgical or legal effectiveness, have little to recommend them from a genetic point of view. Consider first the category of dominant harmful characteristics. Most detrimental dominant genes successfully eliminate themselves from the population. The more harmful it is, the more complete and rapid its elimination. A good example is furnished by retinoblastoma, a dominant malignancy formerly always fatal in childhood. Rare exceptions to this rule resulted from the fact that although retinoblastoma may be exhibited bilaterally, it also occurs unilaterally in a considerable proportion of cases. Hence, with a frequency that is the square of the frequency of unilateral occurrence, it may be expected that a carrier of the gene will escape developing the condition in either eye, and yet will transmit it to half the offspring. By surgical removal of the cancerous eye, a child with retinoblastoma may today survive indefinitely, since the condition does not spread from one eye to the other, but must occur independently in either eye.

Recessive detrimental genes can become far commoner than dominant ones. For example, cystic fibrosis, which is the commonest human recessive lethal condition in Caucasian populations, has an incidence of about one in 2,500 births among American whites. The gene frequency is calculated from this value to be one in fifty, and the frequency of carriers (heterozygotes) in the population is about 4 per cent (Bearn 1972).

Geneticists are deeply concerned about changes in the equilibrium between the introduction of new mutations of a detrimental sort and their elimination from the population. On the one hand are those factors that may increase the mutation rate, such as exposure of the population to larger average doses of ionizing radiation delivered to the gonads, increased exposure to chemical mutagens of many kinds, including most carcinogens, and exposure of the reproductive cells to high temperatures. On the other side of the equilibrium lie all such factors as lessen the rigour of natural selection. Man increasingly makes his environment more controllable and more artificial. Better nutrition, better parental care, and above all else improved medical treatment and prevention of disease, now enable the bearers of once detrimental hereditary traits to survive into the fertile years of life. Hence in ever larger numbers they pass on the once harmful, though now relatively innocuous, genetic defects that occur because of recurrent mutations. We can probably all testify personally regarding the consequences. I, for one, state with proper humility that I am a genetic misfit in at least three ways: I have myopia, allergic sensitivity (severe hayfever) and gout. Probably I have other genetic defects not so evident to myself. Much of my medical history and continuing medical expenses are attributable to these factors. And so it is with most of us. If, in genetic counselling, we are faced with the dread that detection of some genetic defect or carrier status in us will stigmatize us socially, the appropriate response is that everyone in the entire population is indeed in the same boat, though to be sure we are stigmatized in individually different ways.

Constraints imposed by genetics
We would like to eliminate genes that remain strongly detrimental in spite of our best measures, but whatever measures are proposed will fall short, or be objectionable. In the first place, many genetic effects that once were fatal or seriously incapacitating have been rendered innocuous or mild by the application of increasingly better medical and surgical measures to mitigate their effects. For myopia it is easy to obtain glasses; for hayfever, there are antihistamines and desensitization; for gout, colchicine and benamid respectively prevent acute attacks and lower uric acid excretion. Second, it is now evident that some genetic conditions that are harmful in a normal environment may preserve life in other situations. The action of sickle haemoglobin in protecting against malaria is an already classic example. Third, many conditions that are weakening in one environment may be favoured by selection in another. This is probably the case with variations in human skin colour. Fourth, many characteristics interact so strongly with others that their selective advantage or disadvantage is markedly changed. Fifth, many human characteristics of great individual and social importance, such as height, weight, and general intelligence, are determined by the interaction of several or many pairs of genes. True, selection can act effectively upon such characteristics, as is evident from the breeder's success in eliminating multi-factorial genetic defects from breeds of cattle. But artificial selection is possible only when the population can be rigorously controlled in its breeding, and this constraint would be abhorrent to most people.

Positive eugenics
These difficulties have led many geneticists to think that hope lies instead in the direction of positive eugenics, which attempts to encourage

the reproduction of the select. The fallacy of this view has been often disclosed. It is, at least in our time, only fool's gold. For when the same phenotype can be presented to inspection by a large number of different genotypes, and when we commonly do not know the extent to which a character is modifiable by the environment (including pre-natal conditions, childhood nutrition, education and general state of health), there is little way in which we can really identify the ideal or superior person. All the more is this made true by the concealed recessive genes we carry. Probably every one of us carries and may transmit several lethal genes and up to a dozen other quite detrimental genes. Until we can detect the heterozygous condition in respect to far more genetic traits than now, we cannot properly advise or select for eugenic ends.

By far the greatest impediment to positive eugenics, however, is the difficulty in selecting the goals of individual improvement and social evolution. Who is to say what these should be or how they should be combined? Darwin (1871) identified the chief human qualities, in *The Descent of Man,* as 'reason' and 'sympathy'. Muller (1967), apparently quite independently, narrowed down his once large list of desirable goals to two, 'intelligence' and 'cooperativeness'. It is apparent that both thinkers selected the same paramount qualities (Glass 1972c). Intelligence, we know, is inherited to a considerable degree, although we have great difficulty in measuring it or defining it in an unbiased, culture-free way. Even if we could breed successfully for high intelligence, would it be a desirable goal apart from morality and a dedicated social conscience? Who would desire to breed more intelligent criminals? But then are we to suppose that appropriate adjustment to the *present,* so imperfect state of social evolution, with its injustices and denials of self-development and its inequalities of opportunity, should mark the perfect man or woman? Unless we know what the ultimate social order is to be, how can we predict what human types will be best suited for it, or most contented and productive within it?

As for sympathy, empathy, or cooperativeness, no scientific way of measuring them has been attained, and no information as to the degree to which they are heritable rather than conditioned can be presented at this time. Perhaps all we can say with some definiteness is that mankind has achieved its present evolutionary status on the basis of a high degree of genetic diversity, not only interracial but more especially *within* different races and ethnic groups, and therefore that genetic diversity, rather than uniformity, is to be preserved at all costs. That is not only a basis for a plea for greater tolerance of human differences, it stands also as a warning to us not to engage in eugenic programmes the very nature of which is to promote inbreeding and a reduction of human variation.

Euphenics

In the foreseeable future, eugenics, or genetic engineering, will be restricted to the same goals as surgery and medicine (Glass 1972b). Efforts will be expended to remedy the harm done by genetic deficiencies mainly by treating the ultimate symptoms and tertiary consequences. That is what Joshua Lederberg and others have termed 'euphenics', to distinguish it properly from eugenics, inasmuch as such treatment leaves the causal factors, the defective genes, unaltered. As we learn precisely which metabolic step is blocked by a particular inborn error of metabolism and just which constitutive protein or enzyme is deficient in a particular disorder, we can proceed to alleviate the condition in one of two ways. If the disease is thought to result from a lack of the product of the blocked reaction, we can supply that product. If, on the other hand, the disorder is thought to result from the accumulation of the substrate for the blocked step, we can endeavour by means of dietary control, as in the case of phenylketonuria, to reduce the amount of the substrate and its byproducts; or we can remove the diseased or malignant tissue by surgical means, as in the case of retinoblastoma.

Either of these categories of treatment is a symptomatic treatment only. It does not eliminate the cause of the genetic disorder, nor can we by such means prevent transmission of the defective gene to later generations. The first step closer to the root of the trouble would be to operate at the level of the enzyme or primary gene product. That is in most cases impossible by present technologies, because enzymes act chiefly intracellularly, and are either digested when given by mouth or fail to enter the tissue cells when injected into the blood stream. Exceptions to this rule apply only to rather small proteins, such as insulin, which can enter cells, or the immunoglobulins and serum proteins which act in the circulating blood itself.

Genetic engineering

Although future discoveries may surmount these difficulties, the geneticist would prefer to work back to the level of the messenger RNA or the DNA itself. The door to such an achievement seems to have been opened by the discoveries of bacterial transformation and transduction. In the former phenomenon, DNA (deoxyribose nucleic acid), the material of the genes, extracted from virulent pneumococci, can transform a certain number of non-virulent pneumococcus organisms exposed to it into permanently virulent ones. The defective gene in these cases has actually been replaced by the effective allele contained in the extracted (dead!) DNA. In the phenomenon of transduction a supposedly harmless, or latent, virus is used as a carrier of an effective allele from a donor to a recipient possessing only the defective gene. Again, in the bacteria 'transduced', the change is a permanent, heritable one. By promoting entry of the donor DNA into the cells—into the very nuclei—of the second host, the virus makes possible the substitution of the sound gene for the defective one.

In 1971 experiments were reported that indicated a herpes simplex virus had successfully served to transfer a gene for the enzyme thymidine kinase to cultured mouse cells that were genetically deficient for the ability to synthesize that enzyme (Munyon *et al.* 1971). Other workers reported a transformation from galactosemic to normal of human cells growing in culture (Merril *et al.* 1971). (Galactosemia is a human hereditary disorder marked by inability to utilize the galactose coming from digested milk sugar.) Neither of these experiments has been confirmed at present writing, but they point out the way that is being actively explored. It might truly lead to a medical effort to alter the phenotype for particularly severe genetic disorders of metabolism, and would indeed constitute what most persons have in mind when they talk of 'genetic engineering'. What we must remember is that, however successful, such methods would probably leave the defective genes in the reproductive cells of the patient untransformed. Much evidence from cases of mosaic development, in humans as well as other mammals, indicates that the genetic alteration of one organ, whether by mutation, by transplantation, or potentially by transformation or transduction, would not be transferred to other parts of the body.

We thus return to the eugenic dilemma. Whenever a person is restored to reasonable health and survives childhood to enter the reproductive years of life in spite of an inherited disability that would have caused death under the rigours of primitive natural selection, we must reckon with the fact that the treatment fails to change the responsible gene or genes, at least in the reproductive cells. Retinoblastoma and haemolytic icterus illustrate the case for dominant genes. Surgical removal of the eye or the spleen, respectively, is required to save the life of the affected person. Every such person will transmit the dominant gene to one half of the offspring, who will consequently require the same kind of surgical treatment if they are to be saved. Unless the reproduction of such persons is reduced below the ratio for zero population growth (two children per couple), each such case will be followed by another, for all generations to come. This is clearly a way of making more work for future surgeons! It imposes on us the need to provide appropriate genetic counselling and preventive measures.

When the condition is recessive, as in the case of cystic fibrosis or Tay-Sachs disease, every affected person who survives and reproduces will transmit the defective gene to every offspring. The frequency of the gene will consequently rise in the population, although rather slowly, until finally the frequency of affected homozygotes who will need medical care will greatly increase. Some geneticists have dismissed this risk because it is remote. Presumably, by the time many generations have passed, we will have discovered new means of coping with the problem. Maybe so. Yet I must emphasize that what the final frequency will be we cannot foretell. It will differ from case to case, depending upon such further properties as the possible effect of the gene upon fertility, its effect in the heterozygous condition (if any), and its interaction with other genes and with the environment. It is theoretically possible that, in the absence of further selection against the gene, the latter might in time supplant the once normal gene entirely. This is what has happened, somewhere in the ancestry of man, in bringing about our genetic loss of capacity to synthesize vitamin C, an ability which most other mammals retain. The lost capacity necessitates an environment, specifically in the case of vitamin C, a diet, in which the vitamin can be supplied in a regular and sufficient quantity. As long as that can be done, the loss of capacity is no detriment. It might even be regarded as an improvement in some sense, since it frees the organism of any necessity to carry out certain energy-requiring syntheses and spares the substrates for other possible uses.

In other words, although the advances of medicine and surgery in the direction of 'genetic engineering' inevitably increase the burden of defective genes in the human gene pool, they should be classed as detrimental only to the extent of the cost of artificially ameliorating their consequences. At some point, nevertheless, we must cry halt. We cannot blithely accept the possibility of a population in which most persons would require the removal of an eye, or even a spleen. I suggest therefore that a sort of long-term cost analysis is incumbent upon us, a sort of technological assessment of the degree to which we can face with equanimity the prospect of the increasing genetic load that must be controlled by surgery and medicine. The dire alternative would be to apply strong constraints, even to the point of compulsory sterilization, upon persons whose phenotypes we have altered but whose genotypes remain unchanged.

The right to an adequate physical and mental endowment
I have previously maintained (Glass 1971) that in a not-distant future time, owing to the advances of human genetics, the right of individuals

to procreate must give place to a new paramount right: the right of every child to enter life with an adequate physical and mental endowment.

This statement has been frequently misunderstood. I do not argue that some legal body must impose such a right upon reluctant or resistant parents who desire to procreate. I am speaking of a *moral,* not a *legal,* right. When the time comes that prospective parents can through genetic analysis of their own heterozygous genes become fully aware of whatever defects they may transmit as dominant genes, or whatever recessive genes both of them carry in common, and when amniocentesis makes more fully possible prenatal diagnosis of such conditions, we shall enter a new age of moral responsibility in respect to parenthood. Knowledge imposes responsibility and when such knowledge is potentially available, it is morally wrong not to avail one's self of it and to act upon it in the best light of the predictable consequences. The ultimate right to decide, in each individual case, may rest still with the prospective parents, but it will be the obligation of society to provide the fullest information about possible consequences and to give considerate, and at times stern, genetic counsel. In this way, the birth of defective children could be greatly reduced, whether by prenatal diagnosis followed by abortion, or by abstention and adoption of children (or of embryos) of other biological descent. I therefore reiterate that, in a not-distant future, advances in human genetics should make it possible to regard as the paramount right that of every child to be born with a normal, adequate hereditary endowment, one capable of utilizing fully and freely the advantages of equal opportunity in a better society.

References

BEARN, A. G. (1972) Cell culture in inherited disease with some notes on genetic heterogeneity. *New England Journal of Medicine.* **286,** 764.

DARWIN, Charles (1871) *The Descent of Man.* (John Murray: London.) (Second Edition, D. Appleton: New York. 1874.)

GLASS, Bentley (1971) Science: endless horizons or golden age? *Science.* **171,** 23.

—(1972*a*) Human heredity and ethical problems. *Perspectives in Biology and Medicine.* **15,** 237.

—(1972*b*) Genetics and surgery. *Bulletin of the American College of Surgeons.* **57,** 14.

—(1972*c*) Eugenic implications of the new reproductive technologies. *Social Biology.* **19,** 326.

MERRIL, C. R., GEIER, M. R. & PETRICCIANI, J. C. (1971) Bacterial virus gene expression in human cells. *Nature.* **233,** 398.

MULLER, H. J. (1967) What genetic course will man steer? *In Proceedings of the Third International Congress of Human Genetics*. p. 521. (John Hopkins Press: Baltimore.) (Abridged version, *Bulletin of Atomic Scientists*. **24** (March 1968), 6.) Reprinted *In* Bajema, C. J. (ed.) *Natural Selection in Human Populations*. (John Wiley & Sons: New York.

MUNYON, W., KREISELBURD, E., DAVIS, D. & MANN, J. (1971) Transfer of thymidine kinase to thymidine kinaseless L cells by infection with ultraviolet-irradiated herpes simplex virus. *Journal of Virology*. **7**, 813.

CHAPTER 6

Problems raised by eugenics in Africa

John Karefa-Smart

Medical School, Harvard University, Cambridge, Massachusetts, USA

One cf the few generalizations that can be made about the black peoples of Africa is that we place particular emphasis on the predominance of the tribal community and its interests. This emphasis over-rides every other consideration. Questions about what is right or wrong, or good or bad, are therefore properly examined only if this is done within the context of their effects on the tribal community. This is essentially in contrast with the relatively greater importance given to the individual in some other non-African societies.

In black Africa, generally, the tribe is regarded as comprising a tripartite community of three separate segments, namely the ancestors, the contemporary tribesmen and tribeswomen and the yet unborn generations. The first and the last segments have their existence in the spirit world from which they are able, nevertheless, to exert an influence on the middle segment. Everything that the present generations enjoy is a bequest from the ancestors and should be kept and used and passed on, in turn, to the succeeding generations.

In the absence, however, of written systems of thought, we modern Africans, when confronted with contemporary problems, may be tempted to apply the thought systems of the western European nations which have dominated our affairs during the last two centuries; or we may try to seek guidance from the unwritten principles, transmitted by oral tradition, by which we understand that our tribal communities have maintained unity and continuity throughout the past.

Three guiding principles suggest themselves in considering any proposed course of action. These principles may be expressed in the following questions: firstly, is the proposed course of action in accordance with what is known to be the tradition of the tribe as handed on by the ancestors? Secondly, is it likely to be of benefit to the existing community and in its best interests? Thirdly, will it preserve for the succeeding generations the rights to which the legacy of the ancestors entitles them?

Eugenic proposals, I suggest, should therefore be examined from the African point of view by trying to answer these three questions. If Eugenics is a discipline concerned with improving the biological stock of a given population, it would appear, on the surface, that there should be no conflict between the objectives of any eugenic proposal and those of the tribal community which, as has been noted above, seeks preservation, unity and continuity. The possibility of conflict arises when the proposal that is under consideration appears to give paramount importance to the quality of life of individuals and seems to regard the community as essentially a summation of its individuals.

The tribal community, in contrast, regards the individual primarily as an agent through whom the community is able to live and function. Whatever rights belong to the individual derive from his or her relation to the community. Three such rights on which eugenic proposals have a bearing may be mentioned: firstly, the right to procreate or to be the agent of continuity of the tribal community; secondly, the right of the ancestors, under certain circumstances if they so choose, to be reborn or reincarnated; thirdly, the right of the individual and of the community to prevent an intrusion of the world of evil spirits into the community.

Eugenic proposals relevant to these concerns of the tribal community are those designed to regulate individual reproductive capability. These include proposals for selective breeding, and for delayed marriage, proposals for preventing the transmission of undesirable physical characteristics from one generation to the other, and proposals for limiting family size and the total number of individuals in the community.

Certain specific programme activities are usually recommended for the attainment of the objectives of each category of proposal. By examining these objectives in the light of the rights of the individual and the tribal community, and conflicts or potential conflicts should readily become apparent.

Regulation of reproduction may, of course, be proposed for a variety of reasons. Where it is a question of restoring, safeguarding or ameliorating the health of a mother and of her living children, proposals to encourage the use of a variety of forms of contraception present no problems. The objective in these cases is to achieve optimum spacing in the interest of physical, mental and social well-being. If, however, the principal objective is to reduce the rate of population growth for any reasons including eugenic ones, African communities will generally find it difficult to cooperate, because natural increase in the size of the tribal community is implicit in the idea of its continuity. Besides there might be a reluctance to offend the ancestors, because to prevent a given child from being born might be a direct act which thwarts the intention of a departed ancestor to be reincarnated.

Proposals about the practice of abortion, for whatever reason, presents similar difficulties, although we are here concerned only with the advocacy of abortion for eugenic reasons. When miscarriages occur naturally the traditional belief is that some malevolent influence has been at work, and following appropriate rites a new pregnancy is usually sought. It is therefore difficult to imagine that the tribal community will accept a deliberate termination of pregnancy as a desirable practice. It is however difficult to predict how successful health education activities might become in gaining acceptance of scientific ideas such as diagnosis of possible disease in the unborn child by examination of the amniotic fluid. Until these ideas are accepted, advice based on them is unlikely to be heeded.

Infanticide, on the other hand, is not unfamiliar, and is readily advocated or justified under certain conditions in tribal communities. For example when a grossly malformed child is born, it is regarded as a 'devil', and it becomes a duty to prevent its intrusion into the tribal community and infanticide is justified. How far this acceptability can be stretched to cover eugenic considerations it is difficult to predict.

Other examples may be cited, but it is enough to indicate that as far as the African tribal communities are concerned the important consideration is the motive, or the final objective of any proposal, and how this objective affects the community as a whole.

The old beliefs are being given up, however, everywhere in Africa. This is to be expected as a result of encounters with the non-African cultures which appear to be stronger as they are closely associated with the material developments in the towns and cities. Education in western patterned schools, industrialization and migration to the urban communities from the rural areas are all rapidly contributing to a weakening of the bonds of tribal community. The real tragedy would be if new unifying systems of thought and belief do not replace the old ones that are given up. If this were to happen a dangerous void would be created which can only lead to disintegration. It should be the concern of all to preserve integrated community life as much as possible and not subject it to strains by proposals which can not yet easily fit into acceptable traditional beliefs and practices.

CHAPTER 7

Genetic manipulation as a political issue

Kerstin Anér, M.P.

Sweden

The frame of reference for this paper is first of all the industrial countries of the West. Genetic manipulation is a piece of luxury technology and science, which does not concern the developing countries— on the contrary, it may drain resources from problems, the study of which would benefit them much more. The state capitalist countries of the East, also called socialist countries, may be doing some genetic manipulation for all I know, but they certainly have no political discussion going on in this area. Secondly, I am taking for granted that genetic manipulation and engineering is being done, will be done, and may come to be done on a far greater scale and with wider scope than today. I am keeping in mind that several scientists (among whom one could mention Nobel Laureate Jacques Monod, the biochemist) think that any engineering *inside* the gene is something dreamt up by pseudo-scientists and can never become reality. However, what is certainly reality today and almost certainly tomorrow is enough to give any law-giver plenty to think about.

The kinds of genetic manipulation I will consider are: curing of defective genes by treating the genetic material directly; preventing the conception of defective humans by genetic counselling; preventing the birth of defective humans by killing them first.

I will, throughout the rest of this paper, use the common euphemism 'eliminating' for what is done to a foetus that is not allowed to be born. I wish, however, to go on record as stating that there is no known anatomical limit separating the child from the foetus. Even the concept of viability is being continually pressed downward in the age of the foetus. We should know what we are talking about. There may be legal ways of killing, but no way of breaking off a life without killing it. I am going to confine myself to the legal and not the moral issues.

Knowledge and power

The political issue, here as everywhere else, is one of power. Do the new methods of manipulating genetic material and unborn humans confer more power, or new kinds of power, on some people? If so, how should these powers be regulated, curbed, or provided with countervailing powers?

If we look far enough into the future, certainly the power implications of some kinds of genetic manipulation loom very large. A rich country may very well decide to speed up the improvements of its own gene pool by all or any means. But this is rather negligible beside the genetic manipulation that is going on all the time and in the same direction, by conventional means. The children of the rich get proteins during their formative years and so their brains become better than those of their starved or near-starved contemporaries, and a deprived environment lowers the IQ far below that of the children's natural endowments. There is nothing drastically new here, within the next decades at least.

There is another way in which knowledge, as always, gives power; and also, as usual, to those that have, more is given. All experience shows that genetic counselling and screening always interests a sophisticated and well-endowed *élite* of the people much more than those with less knowledge and less affluence. At a meeting in Virginia to discuss genetic counselling in 1971, D. Eaton from All Soul's Unitarian Church, Washington D.C., noted that genetic disease is a much greater preoccupation with whites than with blacks. A positive statement of the same fact can be found in the German book *Menschenzüchtung* (1969), where German jurist Georg Strickrodt writes that he thinks 'broader levels of the population' should be protected from 'psychotic confusion' stemming from too much open discussion on the dangers of genetic manipulation. In his view, only people professionally or idealistically concerned with these questions and qualified to understand them, should be asked for their views, in order to guide the law-givers.

This last view was expressly refuted (although this particular German was of course not known there) at the meeting in Virginia where open discussion was demanded as a minimum necessity for wise public decision-making. This is an issue that crops up all over the place. Who should be allowed to have their say, in matters where professional competence is of the essence in order to get at the facts—yes, even to decide what *are* facts and what are value-judgements? One may quote, for instance, Professor Colin Austin, of the University of Cambridge, an animal embryologist, who deplores the fact that the prospective culture of test-tube babies 'is prone to evoke agitated debate in the press, and emotional pronouncements in high places'. The context makes it clear that the people occupying those invidious 'high places' are bishops, not Nobel Laureates. So some people, according to this authority, are more equal than others when it comes to the right to their own opinions.

A major experiment in mass genetic screening performed so far, the screening for the Tay-sachs disease among around 45,000 Americans of Middle European Jewish descent, has characteristically concerned a fairly well-to-do and educated section of the population. This grows in importance as an indicator of probable future steps when one considers that each and everyone of us carries at least six to eight lethal recessive genes, which means that to eradicate all known genetic diseases equals eradicating all of us. It then becomes a political issue of the highest urgency to decide: what genetic diseases should we try to eradicate, and which should we ignore?

This decision is at the moment being taken by nobody, that is to say by anonymous forces. I am not subscribing to a conspiracy theory in saying this; simply that in a political vacuum other forces rush in. We may not be threatened by Big Brother at the moment, but Big Business is certainly going to come into this area very soon.

Leon R. Kass, Executive Secretary of the Committee on the Life Sciences and Social Policy of the National Academy of Sciences, USA, wrote in 1971: 'we are fortunate that, apart from the drug manufacturers, there are at present in the biomedical area few large industries that influence public policy. Once these appear, however, the voice of "the public interest" will have to shout very loudly to be heard above their whisperings in the halls of Congress.' This applies, in different degree, to all the industrialized countries. It is with a certain lack of enthusiasm that one remembers here the words of one John Platt, who said at a UNESCO symposium in Chichen Itza in 1969: 'I think there could be many billion-dollar pay-offs from million-dollar investments in biological projects in the next few years'. Well, so there may be—but what kind of biology?

It would be naïve to think that no big economic interests are vested in present genetic technologies. The question of whether or not a certain testing programme will show whether a drug causes mutations, means millions not only to the manufacturer of the drug, but also to the manufacturer of the tests. Genetic screening may become a vast medical industry very soon—but how ethical is it to mount important screening programmes, before you know what to do with the people you find defective? And this we do not know, in all too many cases.

Politics and economics

The question of what to do with the human material that is not up to scratch is not only a moral one, but a political and economic one as well. Let me illustrate this with an example from Sweden. This country has one of the most liberal abortion laws in the world, and is actually contemplating liberalizing it even further, perhaps to the limits of 'abortion on demand' (that is, demand by the mother). As soon as this last proposition was being discussed by a Royal Commission, abortion figures (of legal abortions) started soaring to unprecedented heights in Sweden. Not only demand, but the way the health authorities interpreted the letter of the law, was changed by the fact that a new law was being considered.

The Royal Commission put its law project on the table. A violent discussion ensued. The churches of Sweden, and some people, pointed out that the ethical considerations had been simply left aside by the Commission, not even refuted. This made no impact whatsoever. What did make an impact on the Swedish authorities, on the contrary, was the fact that hospitals were swamped by legal abortions and threatened to become even more so, if anything like the new project became law. The new law would have cost millions of crowns to the Health Service (Swedish medicine is to all extents and purposes socialized) and/or would have meant giving less service to women with cervical cancer, for instance. Where the ethical argument failed the economic argument was victorious. The project for a new abortion law was shelved for the present—that is to say at least until after the elections in autumn 1973.

Amniocentesis for genetic screening and subsequent abortion of defective foetuses is thus no legal problem in Sweden. It is, though, an economic one, just like other kinds of abortions. Amniocentesis, in order to find and eliminate foetuses with Down's syndrome (mongolism) and a few other genetic diseases, is being performed in Sweden with very little discussion, but it is impossible to proclaim it a right for every expectant mother, simply because there are not enough geneticists and gynaecologists to go round—and never will be, so the Swedish experts assure me. This means that they concentrate on certain danger groups—for instance, expectant mothers above the age of thirty-five. The doctors engaged in this wish as little publicity as possible, precisely because they cannot satisfy any rising demand. Should they press for the means to do so?

Apart from the moral issues involved—such as the attitude to already existing mongoloid babies, once they come to be regarded as accidents that should not have been allowed to happen—this is one of those political questions that really should be subjected to technological assessment. How much do so-and-so many Down's syndromes cost in an institution, and how much would it cost to train and pay sufficient doctors to track and eliminate them at an early stage? And, as usual, a really satisfactory technological assessment should not stop there. It would have to include something like Leon Kass' questions: are they institutionalized children who have brought the USA into the war in Southeastern Asia? Which group does more harm to the environment during their life-span—mongoloid children, or a year's batch of Harvard students?

There are, of course, other diseases, much worse than mongolism—such as Huntingdon's chorea, and similar horrors—that are also of genetic origin and might be, to a certain extent and in the affluent countries, controlled by amniocentesis and therapeutic abortion. (Or should one say 'social abortion', since it is society no less than the mother who has an interest in it?) Anybody who has seen children and young persons suffering from these plagues will not talk lightly of accepting them as part of nature. Possibly, priorities must be erected here: those diseases we do not accept, that is to say we do not accept persons suffering from them, must have priority over those we find ourselves forced to accept.

I think we must be very much aware of the fact that this is what our choice looks like. It is not just a matter of fighting some benighted obscurantists who want to let people suffer on account of their misguided concepts of human dignity and the value of human life. No—it is far more a question of dollars—what diseases can we afford to fight, and where must we stop, and how do we reconcile our demand for a society uninfested by crocks and invalids, with our wish to respect and help the sick people we cannot just eliminate? Should we retain our respect for the mother, or the family, who prefer to have (or to risk having) a genetically crippled child, rather than eliminating it, or should such mothers be considered in need of psychiatric help?

A young Norwegian Marxist theologian has expressed our dilemma in this way: 'Freedom from the tyranny of nature generally means coming under the tyranny of men. The more technology makes us free from the pressures of nature, the heavier must the social and economic pressure of some people fall on the rest of us.'

Anything we invent that becomes desirable to many persons will become scarce, to a greater or lesser degree, and must be rationed. The allotment may be determined by the purse, or by some *élite* deciding who has the best right to it. This is already a fact in kidney transplantation, while in some countries abortions are the privilege of those who can pay for them or go abroad to have them. Any surgery as complicated as amniocentesis will also always be scarce, and will mean that some people decide—with or without formal political right to do so—who shall get it and who shall not. These are much more urgent questions than setting up a formal, moral fight to one or the other form of surgical help. This is the level at which these questions must be discussed.

Nothing is so futile, when discussing genetic engineering or any other new conquest of science, as talking about 'man' with a capital M and what he is going to do about it. Most men are going to have no chance whatsoever of doing *anything* about it. They will be done to. An example of what I mean is the talk quoted earlier by Professor Colin Austin, where he ends up by saying that banning certain kinds of research—as has been suggested—is a defeatist attitude. 'For if we are to be masters of our fate, we must surely accept the responsibility of exploiting to the full all advances in the control of human reproduction and development.'

Here the keyword is obviously 'responsibility'. But who is responsible to whom? Someone is doing research, other people are being experimented on, and some others, probably rather far away in the future, may be helped by his research. Or again they may not. In this sort of research—on human heredity and reproduction—the excellent ethical rule of doing nothing irreversible, applies with particular force. The stories of DDT and the miracle wheat are there to warn us.

Knowledge and responsibility
In both cases, what looked at first an unmitigated blessing, flowing from the cornucopia of science, proved very shortly to be a mixed blessing indeed. The reason lay in the way the new inventions were used, that is to say, without thought for their real social and ecological consequences. Precisely the same thing is extremely likely to happen when we start raking up the gene pool. We are then meddling with a millenary evolution, whose results may be really known only long after we are all dead. Have we (supposing 'we' could agree on it) the right to decide about what will happen then, on the basis only of our present-day values? We can hardly feel sure we have the right to decide about the hereditary endowment of one single individual, since he can never be asked his opinion about it until after it is far too late. We may assume that he would dislike being born with certain grave inherited defects, that much is true. But since we cannot be sure that we are not putting in something worse, at the same time that we take out something bad, can we really relieve nature of this responsibility and

put it on our own shoulders? Nature is cruel enough. Do we really prefer to suffer for a scientist's mistake than from an 'act of God'? Scientists say today that they must, although reluctantly, play God. Who has asked them to?

One of the reasons why they should *not* play God is that they can't. I should like to quote here at some length what Dr Theodore Friedmann and Dr Richard Roblin (of the Council for Biology in Human Affairs of the Salk Institute for Biological Studies, La Jolla, California) wrote in *Science* on 3 March 1972. Their views have been combated, of course, but I think there is very much to ponder in them:

'For the foreseeable future we oppose any further attempts at gene therapy in human patients because (1) our understanding of such basic processes as gene regulation and genetic recombination in human cells is inadequate; (2) our understanding of the details of the realization between the molecular defect and the disease state is rudimentary for essentially all genetic diseases; and (3) we have no information on the short-range and long-term side effects of gene therapy.

'We therefore propose that a sustained effort be made to formulate a complete set of ethico-scientific criteria to guide the development and clinical application of gene therapy techniques. Such an endeavour could go a long way toward ensuring that gene therapy is used in humans only in those instances where it will prove beneficial, and toward preventing its misuse through premature application.'

Raking up the gene pool has other consequences too. It generally means that we try to abolish certain features of it, parts that we dislike. We hope that the parts left will all be excellent, and evolution will proceed so much the merrier. But evolution doesn't work that way. What has, up to now, been the strength of the human race is its unbelievably varied gene pool kept that way because humans can all interbreed, however long they may have lived apart from each other. It is a well-known fact that as soon as small interbreeding populations are brought into a wider circulation and new genes are allowed to interact with each other, the result is better people—better in the sense of taller, stronger, with fewer hereditary diseases, and in many instances even more beautiful (there are some striking examples here from the Pacific Islands, where many races have met and interbred for a long time). Another fact about the human race, which scientists explain at least partly by referring to the great variation of human genes, is the fact that man alone among the animals inhabits *all* the habitable parts of the globe, and indeed some that you would hardly have thought to be so.

Now, there are some well-known dangers in impoverishing the gene pool of, for instance, domesticated plants. Monocultures, of the same variety of a plant over wide areas, are extremely vulnerable to pests, while cultures of more varied stocks are far less so. At the present moment, we risk losing for ever the ancestral plants from which our present day cereals, etc. were bred once upon a time, and we may thus never be able to breed new kinds if we should need them—as we very probably will. Measures have been taken, not least at the UN Conference on the Human Environment, to stop this depletion and save the gene pools of animals and plants. Should we then start depleting the human gene pools, deliberately, and not knowing what we may be doing to future generations?

There are also projects being broached for improving on our domestic animals, all of which date from the Neolithic breeders we have never been able to supersede. Now, we hope to do so by transferring one or more chromosomes from one species to another. It may soon be possible to do this with mammals, putting a horse chromosome into a zebra or something like that. And of course, people are already beginning to speculate on how to do this to humans.

This is, so far, science fiction, not science. But like all fiction, and especially like all popular fiction, it tells us a lot about how people really feel, and really dream. And we know that once imagination has broken down certain barriers—such as, for example, those separating us from Luna, Mars and Venus—real actions are very likely to follow. And this kind of science fiction says: we need better people, so let us make them better in the laboratory. And what is wrong with that?

Leaving the metaphysical implications aside for the moment, I will simply answer thus: because it means giving an unprecedented power over some people to other people. Let us first set about circumscribing this power, protecting some ordinary human liberties, and then we will see what is left to discuss. The important thing to keep in mind is that being a scientist does not confer on you a moral status superior to that of all mankind so that you need not be accountable for your actions in the ordinary way.

First of all, I would like to exorcise the bug-bear of an international Big Brother, deciding on a global scale what should be made out of all of us. Luckily or unluckily, the nations of this earth will never agree on *anything* to that extent, much less on so controversial a subject as what a perfect human being should look like. Not even a collegium of three dictators, should the earth ever be ruled by such, would be able to agree.

But there are still enough tyrants around, even if on a slightly smaller scale. What is urgently needed in all advanced countries is a legislation on the right to life and limb that is up-to-date and can apply sanctions. The rules about informed consent, to experiments on patients for instance, obviously need tightening up in many countries. When you hear of black patients at a mental hospital in the south of the USA being used as 'voluntary' guinea pigs in experiments where you inject certain chemicals in certain parts of the brain, to produce well-defined changes of consciousness, then you begin to wonder about what 'informed' means in this context.

The rights of the unborn not to be experimented on is something law-givers of hardly any country have yet looked into. But the day is not very far when a doctor may have to decide whether the creature on his laboratory desk is the beginning of a human being, perhaps even a viable one, and as such to be protected by the law like anybody else, although he has no father or mother to look after his rights; or whether it is just a question between the doctor and the sanitary plumbing of the hospital, what is to be done with the thing. Between that day and this, very many experiments will have been done where the laws of the land will be very difficult to interpret, and where the doctor should not really be left absolutely alone to interpret them.

Another legal and moral aspect, which we must grasp without delay, is how the born are to be treated when their sickness or abnormality would be enough to have them eliminated while still unborn. This is now, in some countries at least, left to be decided between the doctor and the parents. It seems to me that we must either say publicly that some human beings simply do not have the same rights and the same dignity as others, or else we must protect those rights. If we will not let a person live unless he/she is 'normal', whatever that means, then we should say so and take the responsibility all together, just as we do in such countries where capital punishment exists, or where we allow a certain amount of persons to be killed on the roads every year, although some quite feasible traffic rules would save their lives.

Laws on how to act in individual cases are not enough, as the last example shows. We also need, as I wrote above, stringent technology assessments wherever we introduce new biological techniques. Such assessments will be very unpopular, especially with politicians. They will entail choosing between saving a few lives by extremely expensive and well-publicized techniques, and saving many or relieving many by dull, uninteresting and personnel-consuming techniques with no lime-light at all. They will also mean choosing between solving social problems by social means, or by medical and biotechnical means. I do not enter into details here—that is a whole new discussion, but much more important than inventing even better and more expensive ways of doing things nobody has ever done before.

This will entail a great deal of hard thinking on what human welfare and genetical welfare really means. It will mean putting a price-tag on every new medical invention. It will mean—alas—putting a price-tag on many human lives. But since this will merely bring to light a practice that is going on all the time, I think it should be done just the same.

This hard thinking should, of course, in great measure be done by professional bodies of the people immediately concerned. The World Ethics Body formed late in 1972 by the Council for International Organizations of Medical Sciences would be a step in the right direction. The extreme power always being laid in the hands of the medical practitioner has always been tempered by the Hippocratic oath and similar codes of ethics, supported by laws wherever possible. This will become even more necessary, as these powers grow to unendurable proportions.

But there is one thing which a body like that will not do, and cannot be asked to do: that is to evaluate the very position of scientific research in society, the value of free research in all and any directions. This must be decided by the people—in the widest sense of the word. *Elites* are good for a lot of things, but not for deciding what *élites* are good for. The sort of questions that science leads us to today touch us all too deeply to be left to the professional answerers of questions.

Take this issue, for instance, proposed by Professor Jean Hamburger of Paris: it is possible that the only way for mankind to survive is to ape nature and use her own drastic, tyrannical and anti-individualistic means. Natural selection has no regard whatsoever for the individual. It is not clear that we can continue to have any such regards when it comes to the right to reproduce, if the race is to survive at all, and in order to make such laws effective, we may have to condition people very drastically in their minds.

To this, an answer comes from geneticist J. F. Crow from the University of Wisconsin Medical School, who points out that at the present level of genetic knowledge in dilemmas pitting individual welfare against the genetic welfare of the species, it is still reasonable to give the benefit of the doubt to individuals. A dialogue like this one (a fictitious one in so far as the speakers do not hear or know of each other, but a real one since they were talking about the same thing) could be duplicated many times all over the world. This is the debate we are all, here and now, embroiled in. And we cannot leave a single human individual out of it because there is not a single individual who will not have to bear the consequences of the answer.

As an end to my own contribution to this debate, I am now going to stick my neck out and baldly put forward what I myself, as a human individual, think:

- A biotechnology for having *more* babies is, at the present moment, a luxury.
- A biotechnology for having *less* babies has a very high priority indeed.
- The matter is complicated, but not decided, by the fact that research on the above two subjects goes hand in hand for a long part of the way.
- A biotechnology for having *better* babies is all right—in principle, but not if it devalues some already existing babies and adults.
- Nor is it all right if it builds on the shaky foundations of what we know today about what 'better' really means.

We may possibly improve on the domesticated animals and plants of the Neolithics—if we are very clever, and have the use of very wide, intact gene pools. But as for improving on Neolithic man—do we know enough? Are we wise enough? I think we should be 'wise enough to know we are not wise enough'.

Experiments that cannot, in their very nature, ever rest on the informed consent of the patient—as in the case of experiments on embryos and foetuses, produced *in vitro* or *in utero*—should no more be considered ethical than experiments on uninformed and involuntary patients in mental hospitals or hospitals for terminal cancer patients. In some countries this will apply only to such embryos or foetuses as risk becoming viable humans, with all those changes in their human nature that the scientist has procured them. In others, it will apply to them even in their foetal stage since they are protected by the laws even then. Any country, however, must reconsider the rights of viable and near-viable foetuses that do not embarrass any mother, preferably before such beings are produced. Afterwards, 'science' may proclaim that it is too late.

PART III

Foetal Diagnosis, Abortion
and Genetic Screening

CHAPTER 8

Foetal diagnosis and selective abortion: an ethical exploration

Roger L. Shinn

Union Theological Seminary, New York, USA

The advance of genetic science presents to mankind new possibilities and raises new ethical questions. This paper concerns only one of these: foetal diagnosis followed by selective abortion. The purpose of this paper is to summarize the main issues in the ethical debates on that possibility in the United States. My own judgments, whether tentative or firm, will undoubtedly colour what I say; but my present purpose is to lift up the most important issues for examination rather than to argue for specific conclusions.

The issues arise because of a new situation for which there are no precise ethical precedents. Foetal diagnosis of some genetic disorders is now possible. Methods include amniocentesis, intra-uterine photography, and use of ultra-sound devices. Of these the most effective method is amniocentesis. This involves the withdrawal, by insertion of a needle, of some fluid from within the amniotic sac inside the uterus of the pregnant woman. Some cells, shed by the foetus, are included in the fluid. They can be examined, usually after growth in a culture. The examination confirms the presence or absence of some—presently only a few—genetic defects. If a genetic abnormality is discovered, abortion is possible.

The seriousness of the ethical issue is obvious. On the one hand, there is the possibility of preventing immense human burdens and sufferings, both of victims of painfully destructive genetic diseases, and of parents and the society that must maintain the victimized lives. On the other hand, this means the destruction of lives because they do not meet the criteria of human worth set by others—an unusual form of medical treatment in that it treats the disease by eliminating the patient.

Some general technical and ethical questions
My aim is to discuss ethical issues, not strictly biological issues. But nowhere is it more evident that technical and ethical questions are not

entirely separable, and the interaction of the two will be obvious in much that follows.

What findings justify abortion?

The practice of amniocentesis generally presupposes that, if a severe foetal defect is discovered, the mother will choose to abort the foetus. In fact, some physicians recommend that no amniocentesis be undertaken unless the mother agrees to undergo abortion in the case of certain findings. Hence the morality of abortion becomes an issue.

In the widespread debates about the morality of abortion, four divergent ethical beliefs recur often:

- Abortion is the equivalent of infanticide. Hence the whole procedure is morally wrong.
- A foetus is not a person and has no moral claim to be brought to birth. Hence the procedure presents no moral problems, but is desirable for the sake of families and societies that will be spared burdens of abnormal children.
- Personhood is conferred neither at conception nor at birth, but is a developmental process extending over a period of time. Hence abortion following amniocentesis is a very serious decision because such an abortion is necessarily a late one—not earlier than eighteen or twenty weeks, which is drawing close to the stage of viability. The United States Supreme Court gives women the right to abortions for any reason in the first trimester. It permits, but does not require, state laws forbidding late abortions unless they threaten the life or health of the woman. Here is legal recognition of the difference between early and late abortions.
- The foetus has *some* moral claim to development and birth, but not an absolute claim against all other considerations. Hence the issue arises of how serious a defect is required to justify abortion—an issue to be discussed further below.

The ethical debate about abortion following foetal diagnosis is not identical with the ethical debate about abortion in general. On the one hand, there are few grounds for abortion stronger than a serious genetic defect. People who have moral objections to abortion sometimes make an exception in this case, feeling that an intensely powerful reason overrides their general moral objection to abortion. On the other hand, a decision to abort a defective foetus may be made far more reluctantly than a decision for an early abortion. Advocates of freedom of abortion usually argue that the minute fertilized ovum is not a person and has few of the characteristics of human selfhood. But abortion following amniocentesis means that the woman has felt the movement

of the foetus within her body; the foetus has a heartbeat and dis-
cernible brain activity; and it is hard to regard impersonally a foetus
when some of its individual genetic qualities are already known. So
some women, who are in general advocates of freedom of abortion on
any grounds, nevertheless believe that abortion in this case requires
grave reasons for its moral justification.

How serious a defect justifies abortion?

Lappé (1973), an experimental pathologist, has stated the issue in all
its moral seriousness. 'What is really at stake is the question of whom
we are ready to admit into the human community.' To this question
there are a spectrum of answers.

One end of the spectrum recognizes few reasons, if any, that justify
abortion because of genetic disorders. This position points out that we
are all defective in one way or another and that the desire for perfect
children is illusory. Only an urgent defect—one that makes meaningful life impossible for the subject and one that puts an overwhelming
burden on family and society—can justify this procedure.

The other end of the spectrum argues that increasing scientific progress will mean that genetically abnormal children will not and should
not be born. Hence even minor defects justify abortion. For that matter,
the preference of parents for a child of a chosen sex is sufficient reason
for abortion of a foetus of the other sex. At least the parents (or
mother) should have the choice, unrestrained by law or inhibitions of
physicians.

Between the two ends of the spectrum are many positions. One
frequent argument, supporting amniocentesis, emphasizes that it can
greatly increase the freedom of some parents. For example, those who
know that the likelihood is one in four that they will produce a child
with a given genetic defect may presently feel morally bound not to
procreate. But, offered the possibility of amniocentesis and abortion,
they may go ahead, knowing that the risk can be circumvented.

An argument for caution about amniocentesis points out that some
of our judgments about desirable heredity are quite uncertain and
sometimes prejudiced judgments. One problematic issue is the XYY
syndrome, of which one geneticist writes: 'The present evidence suggests such individuals are unusually prone to acts of criminal aggression
leading to institutionalization. Until the necessary large-scale surveys
have been completed, it is impossible to say how prone . . . The ethical
dilemma is made the more pointed by the fact that it is not known
whether that extra Y chromosome is directly causal to the difficulties
in which these individuals find themselves.' (Neel 1972.) In this particular case sober scientific judgments have severely criticized early press

reports that influenced popular attitudes about the XYY syndrome.

Wherever a person finds himself on the spectrum of enthusiasm-reluctance for genetic abortion, there are bound to be problematic cases. Hsia (1972) gives an example of genetic disorders that generally affect only males but that may be transmitted by females: 'If one aborts a male foetus with muscular dystrophy or haemophilia, is one justified in permitting a female foetus who is a known carrier of these same defects to come to term so that the problem of diagnosis will repeat itself in the next generation?'

Should amniocentesis be made a routine or even
compulsory practice?
While some would never choose to practice amniocentesis and others would like to see the opportunity widely available, a few would make it compulsory for pregnant women. Their rationale is that certain pre-marital health tests are compulsory in many societies, as are certain tests on new-born infants. Compulsory amniocentesis is comparably justifiable as a way of preventing birth of seriously diseased infants. The rationale assumes either that parents, confronted with clinical evidence of severe genetic defects in the foetus, will choose abortion; or that society has a right to require abortion in some cases on the grounds that parents do not have the right to inflict some defects on children.

The counter-arguments are of two kinds: the 'not yet' and the 'never' positions. The 'not yet' reasoning points out that amniocentesis involves *some* risk (apparently small) to both mother and foetus. Further, the number of disorders discoverable by it is now small. Hence a risk-benefit calculus does not justify it as a general practice, but does justify it in cases where there is reason to suspect discoverable genetic problems; for example, mothers over forty or parents suspected to be carriers of hereditary disease. At some time medical progress may shift the risk-benefit calculus and make mandatory amniocentesis advisable.

The 'never' reasoning says that no woman should be required to undergo abortion, contrary to her conscience or her wish. Compulsion in this area is an intolerable invasion of personal conscience. If she rejects abortion, there is no point in imposing amniocentesis on her.

These debates are a typical case of the way in which judgments combine both technical scientific and more purely moral issues. The risk-benefit calculus is a technical issue that changes from time to time in the light of new information and new capabilities. The question of the meaning of the sanctity of human life and its significance for abortion is a perennial moral issue. So is the question of the relative rights of persons and of society: how far does the individual have the right to resist society's expectations, and how far does society have the moral duty of supporting people whom it judges to be so defective that they should not have come to birth?

Is this procedure a morally dangerous expedient that obscures the more fundamental issue?

It may be argued that the real effort of medicine should be directed toward the treatment of genetic disorders, not the elimination of their victims. Lappé (1973) writes: 'The greatest danger of the institutionalization of prenatal diagnosis is that it will so blunt our moral consciousness that we may forget that a "selective" abortion is only a temporary expedient reflecting our utter helplessness now to deal with the burden of genetic disease'. This statement, as it stands, does not rule out entirely the use of a 'temporary expedient', but warns against any easy institutionalization of it. And the thrust of the reasoning is to put priorities elsewhere.

The counter-argument is that the treatment of genetic disease is difficult, costly, often at present impossible, perhaps in some cases permanently impossible. In any case, for the present, amniocentesis and abortion can reduce human agony.

Whose good is involved?

The importance of this question is that it unveils some rationalizations and requires honesty about motives. Three answers to it are possible.

The first points to the good of the foetus. Some genetic disorders are so severe that it is often argued that abortion is for the good of the foetus. Such a judgment is obviously debatable. Since the foetus cannot be consulted, who is to judge that a damaged life is worse than no life? Are people with Down's syndrome—commonly called mongolism, and probably the most frequent example used in discussions of amniocentesis—really unhappy, if given adequate care? Or do others, who prefer not to have them around, invent this argument to justify their own feelings? What about worse disorders, for example the Lesch-Nyhan syndrome, resulting in mental retardation, compulsive self-mutilation, and usually death in childhood? Would anybody argue that such a life offers gratification to its victim? In a few cases actual law suits have been brought by persons complaining that they should not have been born, although no such suit has been won.

A second answer concerns the good of the parents. The care of a severely defective child can be an overwhelming burden—financial, emotional, otherwise—on parents. Are they morally justified in escaping this burden, especially if the potentialities of the expected child are severely limited or distorted? If parents choose to abort such a foetus, should they honestly recognize that they are making the choice for their own sake? Is moral honesty possible in such decisions?

A third answer emphasizes the good of society. Some diseases require expensive treatment and custodial care. What are society's obligations to pay for such care, and what are society's rights to refuse to do so? Hypocrisy is very easy in such cases. It is easy to talk about the infinite value of every person, while refusing to put out the cash to care for a person. On the other hand, even wealthy societies have limited resources and cannot make possible every conceivable medical treatment for everybody.

Another aspect of the social question is society's stake in the gene pool. Some people, emphasizing personal rights, insist that society may not impose any decisions on the persons most intimately concerned— the parents. An opposing view is stated by Hotchkiss (1973), among others: 'I feel that this gene pool will eventually have to be considered as public property held in common'.

These questions of the good of the foetus, of the parents, and of society are, at best, difficult issues. They are made more difficult by the common human capacity for self-deception in thinking through such questions. The morally important thing is that they not be evaded.

What is the morality of manipulation?
Human procreation began as a natural process, closely allied with the deepest human instincts and vital energies. It took place long before people understood its causes. Increasingly it has come under the dominion of conscious purpose and control. For the most part this is a gain. But people frequently wonder whether, in a technological society, they are abstracting their calculated acts from their inmost natures. Are there points at which our contrived manipulation of ourselves and each other dehumanizes us? To some the attraction of 'natural childbirth', for example, is the recapturing of an inherently human experience that got lost in the apparatus of hospitals and the dulling of consciousness by drugs.

Prenatal diagnosis and selective abortion means an increase in calculation and programming, not a little akin to quality controls in a factory where marred products are rejected. Furthermore, it is a cumulative process. I have already mentioned that it enables parents, who might otherwise refrain from reproduction because they are carriers of genetic defects, to reproduce with the expectation that they can abort defective foetuses. To the extent that this happens, they pass on the genetic problem to the next generation. Pediatrician Judith Hall (1973) calls attention to one consequence: 'This means that those screening programs which are aimed at increasing the quality of our children may, by their very nature, eventually lead to an increasing number of abortions. Procreation will inevitably become more and more of a laboratory science in order to obtain normal babies. Are we willing to pay this price?'

Human manipulation is a polemical term, but its meaning is not precise. Once again, the possibilities can be put on a spectrum. At one end is the idea, apparently feasible, of implanting electrodes in the human organism so as to stimulate pleasure in such a way that the person—if such a being can still be called a person—is titillated into continuous passive ecstasy. Almost anybody finds this dehumanizing. At the opposite end of the spectrum are the simplest uses of drugs or surgery, which can certainly be called manipulation, but which almost nobody finds offensive.

What is not clear is the nature of those acts that intrude, in ethically offensive ways, on human selfhood and human dignity. At what points, in making human life resemble industrial production, does calculation and manipulation isolate humanity from nature in destructive ways? Perhaps nobody can give the precise answer. But ethical sensitivity requires that the question not be suppressed.

What is genetically good and bad?

Every attempt to work with human genetics implies some judgments as to what is good and bad. But at exactly this point some modesty is needed. As Morison (1962) says: 'It is very hard to identify a bad gene. It is even harder to identify good ones.' Dobzhansky (1967) has made the same point: 'Does anybody know what will be best for mankind centuries or millenia hence? . . . No heredity is "good" regardless of the environment'.

On this issue the procedure under discussion, prenatal diagnosis and selective abortion, is a relatively modest one. Although it has grave ethical meaning, because it means the destruction of a foetus at an advanced stage of development, it is not a grandiose program like those which propose to reconstitute the genetic nature of mankind. It aims only to eliminate certain genetic disorders. And it is far easier to identify some defects, with nearly universal agreement that they are defects, than to prescribe desirable genetic futures for mankind. Almost all people will agree that some abnormalities are not desirable in anybody.

Bentley Glass (1971), in a frequently quoted prognosis, says: 'No parents will in that future time have a right to burden society with a malformed or a mentally incompetent child'. The statement, as Glass well understands, bristles with difficulties. Is it conceivable that *all* malformations will ever be eliminated? How serious must malformation be to disqualify a person from life? What means are justifiable to produce this end? Will the elimination of undesirable abnormalities mean also the elimination of desirable potentialities. It is often pointed out that some genes, definitely disadvantageous in some situations, have an advantage for survival and achievements in others.

Genetics is not the only human enterprise that presupposes judgements about what is humanly good and bad. Every political decision, every educational process, every family budget presupposes the same. The difference is that genetic decisions are likely to be irrevocable in ways that other decisions are not. Conceivably future generations might be deprived of valuable opportunities because of superficial genetic judgements in our time. To avoid all judgements of good and bad is both an impossibility and an ethical evasion. A responsible ethic, in making decisions that affect a long future, will remember the fallibility and capriciousness of human judgements.

Is genetics offensively élitist?
The problem is not only that people are unsure of what is genetically good and bad. Often they are too sure. But their assurance reflects their own limited vision. Throughout human history, genetic ambitions (usually in an unscientific or prescientific form) have often reflected the prejudices of racial, social, political, and economical *élites*. The aura of an offensive *élitism* still surrounds much of the literature of genetics.

Kass (1972), a biological scientist, makes the proposition: 'It is probably as indisputable as it is ignored that the world suffers more from the morally and spiritually defective than from the genetically defective'. And Capron (1972), writing from the perspective of the legal profession, says: '. . . our definitions of "disease" and "health" are social as much as they are medical determinations'. If abortion for genetic reasons becomes widely acceptable, only a surrealistic imagination can list the traits that various dictators, scientists, and parents will try to eliminate from future generations.

Yet these very real dangers do not refute the fact that some ailments are recognized with near unanimity as not only undesirable but also intensely painful and destructive of human fulfilment.

Some theological questions
Thus far I have stated several issues which I think almost anybody, regardless of religious commitment, can recognize as important issues. Implicit in them are other issues of special importance to people with

Christian loyalties and theological concerns. The theological questions are not simply additions to the general ethical questions. They involve an intensified probing and sometimes a recasting of the questions that common human experience forces on the agenda.

What is the relation between humanity and nature?
Is nature in some sense a norm for ethics?
One traditional answer, formalized in theories of natural law and natural rights, avows that nature is a norm for ethics. Such an ethic has often been used to oppose 'unnatural' human interventions into natural processes. This style of ethical thinking has been used, often in the past and more rarely today, to oppose contraception, especially by 'artificial' methods. It is sometimes used to oppose abortion. However, its meaning is not unequivocal. It can be argued, in terms of an ethic grounded in nature, that spontaneous abortions are nature's way of eliminating defective foetuses. Deliberate abortions might, by this logic, be simply an extension of nature.

Another answer from the theological tradition affirms that God has given man a creaturely dominion and stewardship over nature. Hence to be human is in some sense both to belong to nature and to transcend nature. It is then part of human dignity to build upon and direct the processes of nature.

By this reasoning, every time people relieve pain or postpone death by improved diet, medication or surgery, they are intervening in nature. All education and culture are an enhancing and constraining of given natural possibilities. To be human is to modify both non-human and human nature.

Even so, within this context, there are rash interventions and violent interventions that constitute an unwillingness to acknowledge human creatureliness. A modest reverence and wisdom will judge interventions with some care, but will not refuse to make them.

How does human dignity affect ethical decision?
Ethical argument about genetics frequently adopts, knowingly or not, the traditional utilitarian calculus. That is, it evaluates any proposal by seeking to reckon its potentialities for increasing pleasure and reducing pain. It may grant that calculations of pleasure and pain are not precise, but they are possible with a rough accuracy. On this basis, amniocentesis, followed by selective abortion, is ethically desirable as a way of eliminating some severe pain and suffering from human life.

In a comparable way, a cost-benefit analysis can be used as a basis for some biological and medical decisions. When limited resources are applied to unlimited needs, the cost-benefit analysis asks where those resources can have the greatest desirable effect. The cost-benefit analysis is sometimes applied in a way that assumes that human valuables are rather easily quantifiable. Garrett Hardin, for example, has reckoned the number of calories invested in a foetus as compared with a human adult; and he has estimated the cash cost of eliminating a defective foetus as compared with enabling it to survive and supporting it through a lifetime. To do him justice, it should be added that he does not limit valuation to calories and cash; he reasons also in terms of psychic and emotional investment involved.

A theological ethic often finds the utilitarian calculus and the cost-benefit analysis offensive. The reason is not that the theological ethic enters the situation with a set of *a priori* commands that resolve issues without empirical inquiry and without any reckoning of consequences. But it does introduce into ethical reasoning a sense of human dignity that skews the methods that rely on quantification.

For example, an experimenter might, without moral qualms, subject plant seeds to radiation in order to increase the number of mutations, either for the pure acquisition of knowledge or with the hope that a tenth of a per cent of the mutations would be valuable and the rest could be thrown out. That might be a profitable cost-benefit procedure. An experimenter cannot morally do that to people. Human dignity intrudes on the calculus.

The illustration shows that the sense of human dignity, inherent in a theological ethic, is widely shared in many types of humanistic ethic. It may be that the peculiarly theological component is what is traditionally called the 'alien dignity' of man. This doctrine suggests that human dignity, far from being easily recognizable, is often hidden and distorted. It is less a human achievement and claim than a divine bestowal. For this reason, a theological ethic often maintains that God's special love for the weak and defenseless requires of persons a comparable concern for the abnormal and those likely to be rejected by society.

Faith does not, of itself, deliver pre-determined answers to human perplexities, including those new perplexities introduced by scientific innovations. It does propose a context of decision that modifies or even upsets simpler conventional moral evaluations.

Can deterministic processes be guided by free moral decisions?
A paradox of determinism and freedom seems to run through almost all attempts to improve human life. It has analogies to traditional theo-

logical debates, but is recognizable apart from them. It may be stated in two propositions:

- All science, including healing science, assumes some causal determination. Do this, and certain consequences are predictable or at least probable.
- The same science assumes some freedom on the part of the agent who rationally and purposefully chooses to initiate causal processes for the sake of expected consequences.

The paradox is one of those perennial puzzles that haunts intellectual history, and it is not likely to be smoothed out suddenly in this generation. But some clearly fallacious answers can be unveiled. Among these, the most dangerous is that answer which assumes that an experimenter or manipulator is doing a rational, purposeful, moral act upon a human object who is only a physico-chemical mechanism. Whatever human transcendence of mechanical processes is ascribed to the agent must have some relevance for the human object.

If a geneticist is simply carrying out the coded instructions of his own genetic constitution, with no capacity for making judgements that in any sense transcend his own programming, there is something ludicrous in the whole notion that he is intentionally aiming at some good. Yet if there is something of genuine freedom in persons, there must be points at which such freedom demands respect.

In standard medical practice such freedom is acknowledged in the principle of informed consent. This is often a perplexing principle to put into practice. It runs into special difficulties in the case of the foetus, who cannot give informed consent to anything, including its own birth or destruction. Yet if consent is totally irrelevant, genetic practices are morally precarious.

The ethical issues involved in the new genetics deserve the most thoughtful continued discussion, for two reasons. First, their intrinsic importance is great, inasmuch as they involve decisions that may affect the human future on a momentous scale. Second, they are paradigmatic examples of the human encounter with decisions for which there is little or no precedent in ethical traditions.

This generation of mankind lives in a situation where it cannot see in advance the shape of human life a few generations hence. We can, however, be almost certain of the need for an ethic of exploration.

References
CAPRON, A. M. (1972) Genetic therapy: a lawyer's response. *In* Hamilton, M. (ed.) *The New Genetics and the Future of Man*. p. 133 (Eerdmans Pub. Co.: Grand Rapids, Michigan.)

DOBZHANSKY, Th. (1967) Changing man. *Science.* **155,** 409.

GLASS, Bentley (1971) Science: endless horizons or golden age? *Science.* **171,** 23.

HALL, Judith (1973) The concerns of doctors and patients. *In* Hilton, B., Callahan, D., Harris, Maureen, Condliffe, P. & Berkley, B. (eds.) *Ethical Issues in Human Genetics: Genetic Counseling and the Use of Genetic Knowledge.* Fogarty International Center Publication Proceedings No. 13. p. 23. (Plenum Publishing Corp.: New York.)

HOTCHKISS, R. (1973) Discussion. *In* Hilton, B., Callahan, D., Harris, Maureen, Condliffe, P. & Berkley, B. (eds.) *Ethical Issues in Human Genetics: Genetic Counseling and the Use of Genetic Knowledge.* Fogarty International Center Publication Proceedings No. 13. p. 19. (Plenum Publishing Corp.: New York).

HSIA, D. Y. Y. (1972) Detection of heterozygotes. *In* Harris, Maureen (ed.) *Ethical Problems in Human Genetics: Early Diagnosis of Genetic Defects.* Fogarty International Center Publication Proceedings No. 6, DHEW Pub. No. (NIH) 72-25. p. 15. (National Technical Information Service, US Dept. of Commerce.)

KASS, L. R. (1972) New beginnings in life. *In* Hamilton, M. (ed.) *The New Genetics and the Future of Man.* p. 15. (Eerdmans Pub. Co.: Grand Rapids, Michigan.)

LAPPE, M. A. (1973) How much do we want to know about the unborn? *Hastings Center Report.* **3:1,** 8.

MORISON, R. S. (1962) Comment. *In* Hoagland, H. & Burhoe, R. W. (eds.) *Evolution and Man's Progress.* p. 63. (Columbia University Press: New York.)

NEEL, J. V. (1972) Ethical issues resulting from prenatal diagnosis. *In* Harris, Maureen (ed.) *Ethical Problems in Human Genetics: Early Diagnosis of Genetic Defects.* Fogarty International Center Publication Proceedings No. 6, DHEW Pub. No. (NIH) 72-25. p. 219. (National Technical Information Service, US Dept of Commerce.)

CHAPTER 9

Ethical problems in foetal diagnosis and abortion

Barbara H. Sanford

*Department of Microbiology,
Harvard School of Public Health, Boston, Massachusetts, USA*

Until recently, efforts at prevention of genetic disorders have been directed largely at identification of high risk families and at counselling them concerning the probability of their having affected children. Now, development of methods for cytogenetic and biochemical analysis of cells cultured from fluid withdrawn from the amniotic sac during mid-pregnancy has made possible prenatal diagnosis of many genetic disorders (Emery 1970; Carter 1972). Combining this approach with selective abortion of defective foetuses provides an opportunity for preventing the birth of many severely defective children and thus reducing the immediate burden to the family and society. On the other hand, there are some very real problems—biological, social and ethical— related to the use of these procedures.

Risk to the mother

There is considerable divergence of opinion concerning the risks involved in foetal diagnosis and selective abortion. Risks to the mother from amniocentesis (the procedure currently used most often for foetal diagnosis) include haemorrhage, infection, spontaneous abortion and blood group sensitization (Fuchs 1972; Nadler 1971). Although there is no question that such complications can occur, the degree of risk has been assessed differently by various investigators. Milunsky *et al.* (1972) recently reported a very low rate of maternal complications in ninety-four pregnancies studied at the Massachusetts General Hospital. They concluded that the procedure was relatively safe and urged obstetricians to consider indications for amniocentesis for genetic disorders in every patient. On the other hand, Nadler (1971) after summarizing results of four groups using amniocentesis in a total of 370 pregnancies cautioned, 'Because of the risks involved and the consequences of the results, only people with a great deal of experience should undertake amniocentesis'.

There are, of course, additional risks when a decision is made to terminate a pregnancy. Because successful amniocentesis can rarely be performed prior to the fourteenth week of pregnancy, abortions are generally done during the second trimester. As pointed out by Fuchs (1971), abortion at this time is much more traumatic to the mother than early abortion, both physically and emotionally.

Risk to the foetus

Dangers to the foetus from amniocentesis include death, damage or infection (as a result of insertion of the needle into the amniotic sac) and abortion induced by the trauma of the procedure. Published studies so far suggest that the rate of such complications is low. On the other hand, as several investigators have cautioned, there is at present limited data even about immediate risks, and it is still too early to determine whether a foetus subjected to this procedure may show subtle damage in later life. It should be remembered that in most cases the foetuses under study will be found unaffected, and one questions the extent to which the normal individual's well-being can be jeopardized in attempts to detect the abnormal.

Reliability of diagnosis

Errors in diagnosis can of course be in either direction. In some cases an affected child has been born although the defect had not been detected in the cells studied, with resulting emotional shock to the parents involved who had mistakenly been reassured about the expected outcome of the pregnancy. In the reverse situation, some normal foetuses have been aborted as a result of 'false positive' test results.

Most workers agree that reliability of the procedure in detecting gross chromosomal abnormalities is high, provided that an adequate cytogenetic laboratory is available to perform the analysis. On the other hand, diagnosis of metabolic disease is more difficult and after reviewing the experience of several groups, Nadler (1971) recently cautioned, 'Despite the advances in the past few years, a great deal more experience is required before amniotic fluid, uncultured amniotic cells and cultivated amniotic fluid can be used as a routine method for the antenatal detection of familial metabolic disorders'.

Genetic effects

Most cases of gross chromosomal abnormality occur sporadically, with affected individuals having low viability and reproductive capacity; thus their removal at a prenatal stage would be expected to have little effect on the genetic structure of the population. An exception occurs however, with 'balanced translocation', which is estimated to occur in at least three per 1,000 adults in human populations (Hamerton 1969). Here an apparently normal individual has a deletion of part of one chromosome and a corresponding amount of excessive material on a chromosome of another pair, and familial transmission is seen.

Because the translocation itself can lead to disordered meiosis and because gross chromosomal imbalance may lead to loss of germ cells or early undetected abortion, there is no simple formula for calculating the expected percentage of affected offspring. As Hamerton (1970) has pointed out, the frequency of defective children with unbalanced chromosal constitutions from carriers of balanced translocations is in practice 'much lower than the theoretical 50 per cent'. On the other hand, Ford and Clegg (1969) have reported that among phenotypically *normal* offspring of individuals with a balanced translocation, there is a significant increase over the 50 per cent expectation for carriers of the balanced translocation, with approximately 60 per cent of apparently normal offspring studied being carriers.

With the availability of prenatal diagnosis and selective abortion, the risk of bearing a chromosomally unbalanced defective child can be replaced by the risk of undergoing a mid-term abortion. To whatever extent the carriers of balanced translocations are thereby encouraged to have more children, the frequency of chromosomal abnormalities in the population will be increased, since at least half of the offspring, although themselves unaffected, will carry the balanced translocation. It has been suggested that the detrimental effect on the population could be avoided by aborting carriers of the balanced translocation (Miller 1971). Could one morally justify aborting a clinically normal foetus solely on genetic grounds? Even if this were considered acceptable, one would wonder how a mother would tolerate such a high risk of having each pregnancy end in abortion.

As Neel (1972) has pointed out, a similar situation occurs with X-linked or autosomal recessive genes with deleterious effects. To whatever extent the availability of foetal diagnosis encourages the carriers of a deleterious gene to increase their families, the population frequency of the deleterious gene involved will rise. (This occurs because if affected offspring are aborted half of the female offspring in the case of an X-linked recessive disorder and two-thirds of all offspring in the case of an autosomal recessive, although themselves normal, can be expected to be carriers of the deleterious gene.) Although there seems to be no debate among geneticists that this dysgenic effect will occur, there is some controversy about its magnitude and significance. Motulsky *et al.* (1971), for example, examined the effect of selective abortion on the frequency of genes causing autosomal recessive diseases and concluded that the overall effect would be trivial. Hagy and Kidwell (1972), on the other hand, pointed out that the effects of continued mutation had not been taken into account in these calculations and, after re-examining the issue, concluded that the ultimate effects could be substantial. Certainly the extent to which we should attempt to alleviate the burden of genetic disease today by adding to the genetic burden of future generations is an ethical question of major proportion. Aborting carriers as well as affected offspring seems a poor solution, since all of us are carriers of some hidden deleterious genes and it would be difficult morally to justify elimination of normal individuals who carry certain genes which happen to be detectable.

Aside from the dysgenic effects of selective abortion, another ethical problem arises in cases of those X-linked disorders which cannot be diagnosed prenatally. In such cases, abortion of all male foetuses is often proposed. One would certainly question the morality of aborting all males in this situation, knowing that half of them are expected to be normal.

Only when a disorder shows dominant inheritance and thus is recognized in heterozygotes could we expect to reduce the gene frequency in the population by selective prenatal elimination of affected individuals. At the moment this possibility has little impact since there are no dominantly inherited genetic disorders which can presently be reliably diagnosed in prenatal life.

Other aspects

Other problems related to prenatal diagnosis and abortion may be profound and are just beginning to surface.

Very little, for example, is known about the psychological and social effects of such procedures upon the family (which in these cases often includes at least one severely defective child). How does the family tolerate the stress of second trimester abortion? Might a mother who really did not want to undergo pregnancy under these conditions feel guilty about her decision? What might be the effects upon an abnormal child already present in the family and upon his siblings? (Might he perhaps wonder about his own right to live or about his parents' attitude toward him as reflected by their unwillingness to risk another affected child?)

If, as Nadler (1971) suggests, these procedures should be carried out only where appropriate medical experts are available, will a large segment of the population be supporting (perhaps indirectly through insurance premiums or taxes) an expensive service available only to those living near major medical centres? If the procedures have value, should they not be made widely available, perhaps as part of public health programs?

What are some possible legal complications? Are there legal questions concerning the rights of the foetus? What if parents disagree as to what course to follow?

Are there dangers of misuse of such techniques for political or social reasons? If so, what precautions should be taken to guard against this?

While most of us would perhaps agree that the parents involved should make the ultimate decision about pregnancy termination, we are all aware that such a decision is not made in a vacuum but is affected by information and advice provided, by previous experience, and by the whole cultural and social milieu. Where are parents to turn for counselling, not only for medical and genetic information but for advice on psychological, socio-economic and spiritual aspects of the problem? To what extent should the good of society—present or future—be taken into account if it appears to be in conflict with the good of the individual?

Clearly there are many issues involved which are more social or ethical than medical; hopefully these will receive much thoughtful consideration (particularly from such interdisciplinary groups as this particular consulting panel) before decisions are made about wide-spread use of foetal diagnosis and selective abortion.

Acknowledgements

I wish to thank Professors Herman B. Chase, George W. Hagy, James F. Kidwell, and Dr Ann M. Chase of Brown University, Providence, Rhode Island and Professors Roger L. Nichols and H. S. Salhanick of the Harvard School of Public Health for constructive comments on the manuscript.

References

CARTER, C. O. (1972) Practical aspects of early diagnosis. *In* Harris, Maureen (ed.) *Ethical Problems in Human Genetics: Early Diagnosis of Genetic Defects.* Fogarty International Center Publication Proceedings No. 6, DHEW Pub. No. (NIH) 72-25. p. 17. (National Technical Information Service, US Dept. of Commerce.)

EMERY, A. E. H. (1970) Antenatal diagnosis of genetic disease. *In* Emery, A. E. H. (ed.) *Modern Trends in Human Genetics.* p. 267. (Butterworth: London.)

FORD, C. E. & CLEGG, H. M. (1969) Reciprocal translocations. *Biological Medical Bulletin.* **25,** 110.

FUCHS, F. (1971) Amniocentesis and abortion: methods and risks. *Birth Defects: Original Article Series.* **7,** 18.

—(1972) Amniocentesis: techniques and complications. *In* Harris, Maureen (ed.) *Ethical Problems in Human Genetics: Early Diagnosis of Genetic Defects.* Fogarty International Center Publication Proceedings No. 6, DHEW Pub. No. (NIH) 72-25. p. 11. (National Technical Information Service, US Dept. of Commerce.)

HAGY, C. W. & KIDWELL, J. F. (1972) Effect of amniocentesis, selective abortion and reproductive compensation on the incidence of autosomal recessive diseases. *Journal of Heredity.* **63,** 185.

HAMERTON, J. L. (1969) Reciprocal translocations in man. *In* Darlington, C. D. & Lewis, K. R. (eds.) *Chromosomes Today.* Vol. 2. p. 21. (Oliver and Boyd: Edinburgh.)

—(1970) Foetal sex. *The Lancet.* **1,** 516.

MILLER, O. J. (1971) Discussion of symposium papers. *Birth Defects: Original Article Series.* **7,** 33.

MILUNSKY, A., ATKINS, L. & LITTLEFIELD, J. W. (1972) Amniocentesis for prenatal genetic studies. *Journal of Obstetrics and Gynecology.* **40,** 104.

MOTULSKY, A. G., FRASER, G. R. & FELSENSTEIN, J. (1971) Public health and long-term genetic implications of intrauterine diagnosis and selective abortion. *Birth Defects: Original Article Series.* **7,** 22.

NADLER, H. L. (1971) Indications for amniocentesis in the early prenatal detection of genetic disorders. *Birth Defects: Original Article Series.* **7,** 5.

NEEL, J. V. (1972) *In* Harris, Maureen (ed.) *Ethical Problems in Human Genetics: Early Diagnosis of Genetic Defects.* Fogarty International Center Publication Proceedings No. 6, DHEW Pub. No. (NIH) 72-25. p. 219. (National Technical Information Service, US Dept. of Commerce.)

CHAPTER 10

An ethical view of abortion *

André Dumas

Protestant Faculty, Paris, France

There are two ways of doing ethics. We can start from universal and unalterable objective principles or we can start from particular and variable subjective situations. Each approach has its advantages and disadvantages. Let me indicate these advantages and disadvantages briefly and frankly. An ethic of general principles reminds the individual of the best that is required of him in the absolute sense. It does not vary with time or place. It is independent of scientific discoveries, population statistics and opinion polls. It sticks to the essential values and strives to maintain these values, 'come wind, come weather'. But an ethic of general principles can all too easily become cold and abstract, which in human terms means insensitive, merciless and oppressive. It then turns into a law, inducing agonies of guilt and loneliness instead of helping people really to live. An ethic of general principles can even be demoralizing when it is common knowledge that its principles are not practised, yet these principles continue to be reasserted long after they have forfeited all credibility. People then begin to question whether such an ethic is really based on true values or, at least, whether it is capable of adequately expressing these values.

A situational ethic, on the other hand, considers each specific case, trying to grasp its logic, to discern its motives, to go along with the hopes invested in it. It does so to such an extent, however, that it may well be asked whether it is still, strictly speaking, an ethic at all, in the sense of a claim and a responsibility as well as in the sense of reassurance. Is it not simply an endorsement of the morality which has actually developed up to this point? The danger is that, in its anxiety to avoid any appearance of legalism, it may engender a new kind of loneliness, the loneliness of individuals left entirely to their own reactions without any question arising of good or evil in what they do. In that case, the various forms of situational ethics also have a demoralizing effect, suggesting, as they seem to do, that moral choice is henceforth

* Translated from French

eliminated by the development of technology and social customs, and simple solutions are now available to the extent that we can now inter-vene in processes which hitherto were seldom tampered with, either because of inadequate knowledge or for fear of a thunderbolt from on high.

True morality, as I see it, is based neither on abstract general prin-ciples nor on accurate descriptions of actual situations, but rather on conflicts. Moral problems arise where there is a conflict between values equally worthy of respect, where we are not sure which should take precedence and find ourselves up against profoundly difficult and comp-licated questions, where we find it impossible to entrench ourselves behind general principles or simply let each situation take its natural course. Today more than ever, abortion is a moral issue of this kind: a source of conflict, a matter of urgency, a cause of uncertainty.

Abortion is, moreover, only one example—undoubtedly the one met most frequently among all the peoples of the world—of the crucial contemporary problem of man's interference with life, that is with physical nature itself, bearing in mind the root meaning of *phusis* which denotes 'life' itself and not inanimate realities (*phusis* comes from *phuein* 'to grow'). In the Bible, man's intervention in the life of the living world around him is described as part of the divine promise to man. According to the priestly liturgy of creation: 'God (*Elohim*) blessed them' (that is man, male and female) 'and God said unto them, Be fruitful and multiply, and replenish the earth, and subdue it: and have dominion over the fish of the sea, and over the fowl of the air, and over every living thing that moveth upon the earth.' (*Genesis* 1:28). According to the Yahwistic account of creation, man's intervention is a task assigned him by God: 'the Lord God (*Yahweh-Elohim*) took the man and put him into the garden of Eden to dress it and to keep it.' (*Genesis* 2:15).

Since from the Biblical standpoint nature and life are not divinities requiring man's worship and obedience but rather gifts of God to be used and cared for by man, man's intervention in this natural area is something promised and therefore at the same time permitted and commanded. The desacralization of life is thus the prelude to its sancti-fication. When we believe that life, having its goal in God, is not 'sacred' (in the sense of being the receptacle of an immanent and name-less divinity, in the sense of an inviolable taboo), intervention in this natural sphere is possible. Indeed we must do so, since we are to 'till' it and 'care for' it, and this means neither neglecting it nor destroying it. Desacralization in its proper form leads to the sanctification of life, not to its manipulation.

Man's dominion over nature

Man's achievement of this dominion over animate nature actually takes place in two successive stages: first, man's dominion over the animal world; next his dominion over the life of man. The Biblical texts were, of course, written while man was still in the first of these stages. But I believe we can still learn from these Biblical passages today at a time when the great biological revolution is carrying us over the threshold of the second stage. According to the Bible, God in His goodness offers to man an environment consisting of the living creature (literally that which has a 'living soul'), not only the wild 'beasts' of the earth but also the domestic 'cattle' (*Genesis* 1:25-26). This blessing bestowed on man by God has a liberating effect, enabling man to conquer any fear of the animal because of its supposed 'sacral' character. This desacralization of the animal world is accompanied, however, by a series of very detailed sanctification rites, designed to remind man that the animal life by which he is nourished is still a life given by God and not a life of which he is to become either the supreme lord or the infatuated devotee. The Old Testament, especially in its priestly traditions akin to the first creation narrative, distinguishes between clean and unclean animals, between those which may be consumed and those whose flesh man is forbidden to eat (*Leviticus* 11). Although it is not easy to understand fully the origin of these terms, their exhortatory purpose is clear enough. God allows His people a share in the use of this animal kingdom. At the same time, by imposing certain ritual obligations, He reminds them that the animal kingdom inhabits God's own dwelling place, lives on this earth sanctified by Him, lives within the creation He makes holy. This reminder is in the form of prohibitions, just as in the garden of Eden man was permitted to eat from every tree except the tree of the knowledge of good and evil. 'I am the Lord your God: ye shall therefore sanctify yourselves, and ye shall be holy; for I am holy: neither shall ye defile yourselves with any manner of creeping thing that creepeth upon the earth. For I am the Lord that bringeth you up out of the land of Egypt, to be your God: ye shall therefore be holy for I am holy.' This then is the law concerning beast and bird, every living creature that swims in the water and every living creature that teems on the land. It is to make a distinction between the clean and the unclean, between living creatures that may be eaten and living creatures that may not be eaten (*Leviticus* 11:44-47).

The transition from the Old Testament to the New is marked, of course, by the abrogation of these food regulations, since, unlike the Jews, Christians believe that Jesus Christ is the final and supreme priest who came to fulfil and complete the significance of these distinctions between clean and unclean by being himself the one who desacralizes and sanctifies the whole earth. Nonetheless, the Old Testament continues to point us in the right direction as mankind acquires the cultural and scientific means of intervening in the very life of man himself. In this new dominion, too, we must discover a way whereby life itself is not turned once again into a false god, a way which does not however at the same time leave human life entirely at the mercy of unrestricted and uncontrolled experimentation, as if man were the sole master of the world of living things. If ancient Israel had to face the problem of formulating distinctions in the form of exhortations in respect of the animal kingdom, how much more necessary this is today in respect of man himself, created in the image and likeness of God, that is like God Himself, a unique person, whereas the Bible always refers to the animal as a 'kind', a 'species', 'teeming' in the different environmental elements of the universe (the word 'kind' occurs no less than six times in verses 21, 24 and 25 of *Genesis* 1). It may confidently be affirmed that the distinction we need to make here is that between 'life' and 'person'. Life is offered to man as a domain in which he is at liberty to intervene both by his researches and by his practical action. It would be arbitrary to distinguish here between human 'life' and animal 'life'; there is no spiritual basis for or scientific truth in such a distinction, ignoring as it does the contiguity and continuity of these two forms of 'life' as both the Bible and science testify. There is no reason for us to be afraid, therefore, of the advances in contemporary biology which now make it possible for man to intervene in the genetic processes, to carry out transplants, to plan improvements, and even to advise against impregnation in certain cases. We must learn to accustom ourselves to such interventions without being afraid of them, just as ancient Israel received 'theological' permission to make use of the animal kingdom, the world of living creatures, for food. On the other hand, the human person is not at the disposal of another human person, since the human person belongs strictly to God, who knows and sanctifies it.

Man's dominion over men

As we are only too painfully aware in our contemporary world, torture is the attempt to bring one human being under the dominion of another human being by the infliction of pain. Exploitation and destruction here take the place of sanctification. But there are less extreme cases where the question of violation of the human person arises, as distinct from the question of respect for life itself. I include here all those instances where intervention takes place contrary to the express will or implicit desire of those who are its objects, where the latter are in no sense treated as responsible subjects. On the other hand I also include all the cases where the outcome of failure to intervene would be human lives having practically no possibility of development as persons; all those cases where pure scientific curiosity takes precedence over human concern for persons; and finally—and this certainly needs saying—I also include all those cases where techniques and resources are so concentrated on particular persons that it is impossible for help to be given in other personal situations, situations where decisive results could be achieved with a much more modest concentration of such techniques and resources.

This distinction between, on the one hand, life itself as desacralized, and on the other hand, the human person intended for sanctification, is not an easy one to make. The human person is bound up with and present in the life of the body. It is impossible for us, therefore, to speak of it as if it were located elsewhere, as if it were a late arrival on the scene or as if it departed earlier, in the way that ancient Greek anthropology (which is not the same as the Biblical) used to speak of the soul arriving subsequently to 'animate' the body distinct from itself, from which the soul is able to 'escape' as the discarded fleshly envelope disintegrates in corruption.

Apart from the physical life, therefore, there is no person, and, by the same token, there is no physical life to which we could deny the presence of all personal quality. We cannot, therefore, resurrect the ancient dualism in a new form by replacing the ancient dualism of soul and body with a dualism of person and life. Nevertheless, the distinction between person and life, which could not possibly be made between entities assumed to be utterly alien the one to the other, remains a fundamental one for both the scientist and the theologian in the pursuit of their different goals. Life itself is there for the sake of the person, not the person for the sake of life. A personal existence is not to be sacrificed, erased, or forgotten, in some way or other, for the sake of life itself. The very extent of our power to intervene in life itself, today involves us all in new conflicts of conscience, in the medical, political and social fields. How will interventions of this kind help us to achieve a more effective service of persons, a greater respect for persons? As we enter on this second stage of the desacralization of animate nature, how can we make it one which helps to promote the sanctification of persons and prevent it from degenerating into impersonal manipulation? Are there any political guidelines we could suggest here and does the Judaeo-Christian tradition provide any resources which could be useful to us here?

Intensification of moral conflicts in connection with abortion

Let me begin with the advance in medical techniques. Medical practice is becoming ever more successful in protecting life from the threat of death. Where nature is frail, ailing or defective, medical science is able to intervene to correct it. Medical science enables human beings to live on and survive despite infirmity, especially in infancy and old age. It saves and heals. But the very progress it has made in this direction leads it to an ever deeper understanding of the different stages of human growth from the very moment of conception, and consequently increases its capacity to intervene. For example, it is now possible to detect possibly abnormal developments much earlier and with much greater certainty. Medical science also reduces the physical and psychological risks of such intervention. By making it easier it diminishes the element of drama. Medical progress has two consequences, therefore, and there is a growing tension between them. Not only are we in a better position to protect life, we also know more reasons for interrupting it and, if we need to do so, more methods of accomplishing this. Knowledge of how to save life goes hand in hand with knowledge of how to terminate it. We need only picture to ourselves the hospital with its resuscitation unit and its abortion unit side by side in the same building to have an eloquent reminder of the dual contribution made by the progress of one and the same science.

A similar picture presents itself when we consider the whole vast area concerned with the reception of the infant from a psychological and pedagogical standpoint, taking these terms in their widest sense. Modern society obviously pays much more attention to this than did its predecessors. It is generally recognized that the introduction of a human infant into the world takes much longer than the time required for its biological delivery from its mother's womb. Emotionally, socially, culturally, economically, in so many ways, the human infant is born prematurely. Welcoming an infant means, therefore, providing it with a living active environment lasting long enough and of such a kind that it will make it possible for the infant to become the human being for which its biologically complete substratum provides no more than the potential. Modern progress in the reception of the infant at once raises the question of possible medical intervention when the immediate or long-term prerequisites for this reception appear to be completely absent. Modern thinking on the question of abortion should not be dismissed, therefore, as hostile towards the infant. On the contrary, it is very often the advance of scientific understanding which underlines this thinking; for example, the psychoanalyst's insight into the importance of the child's being wanted, the educationalist's insight into the educative potentials, and so on.

The same paradoxical aspects confront us when we consider the field of demography. Individually as well as at the family, national and world levels, we have come to realise that the limitation of natural fertility is a necessary, legitimate and beneficial step, and that this suggests the use of birth control methods. Now, however, in view of the relative inadequacy of the various methods of birth control and of the discipline they presuppose, the question arises whether abortion ought not to be openly included as another possibility when birth control has failed (or, more often, if truth be told, simply not been tried) especially since abortion has in any case always been used, with varying degrees of concealment, as a method of controlling the number of unwanted births. As with advances in medical science and with the reception of the infant, so too the population explosion has two aspects: on the one hand more and more lives are saved, but on the other hand increasing provision is being made for the termination of lives.

The outcome of these various factors is a change in our attitude to life, or rather a dual approach to it from two different standpoints which come increasingly into conflict. From one standpoint life is affirmed as a supreme value, always to be defended and especially so perhaps when it is unable to defend itself. This is the standpoint automatically adopted and respected in professional medical ethics. It is the standpoint of the great religious traditions and of legal codes which make it an offence to injure our fellow men. From another standpoint, however, life is not a biological function which can be treated in isolation from the total context of its future development. Life here is not a law of the species but the benediction of the human person. This is why, in the case of human life specifically, quality has to be considered and not merely quantity. Doctors, churchmen and lawyers cannot therefore speak of life as a 'thing' which could exist independently of the people, mainly women, but also men, who will be responsible for providing this life with its proper chance to develop. From this second standpoint, morality does not mean defending life itself as such, but rather fostering it within a whole context of surrounding circumstances, and not declining to intervene, therefore, should these circumstances seem disastrous or even simply inimical, because of being pervaded with regrets rather than feelings of enthusiasm.

I have spoken in very general terms. But my main concern has been that we should appreciate just how sharp are the conflicts and tensions between these two standpoints. Whichever of these standpoints we adopt we should not be too quick to accuse the other of immorality. Both standpoints include authentic values. Precisely for this reason, in my view, all generalizations are false. To prohibit all abortions would not do justice to serious consideration of the importance of environment to a human life. To permit all abortions would not do justice to the equally serious and responsible concern to defend a life which is already biologically complete. A complete ban would surely mean regarding all life as sacrosanct and inviolable. To remove all restrictions would surely be to reduce the act of abortion to a triviality. Does this not mean, then, that we are morally bound to consider individual cases, in such a way that what mankind has gained from new medical skill, from greater heed to psychology and pedagogics, and from sharpened awareness of population problems is not turned into an occasion for irresponsibility or made the basis of a deeper sense of guilt. It should be used as a means of enhancing man's sympathy and of equipping him to support more effectively those who find themselves up against what I still prefer to speak of as a 'boundary' situation. Just as we need to be aware of moral dilemmas and not try to solve them by suppressing one or other of the conflicting elements, so too we must not leave the people who are faced with such a dilemma to wrestle with it on their own. On the contrary we must help them either to solve it by a deliberate and voluntary act or else to come to terms with it by an equally deliberate and voluntary acceptance. Morality means an increase in responsibility. A total ban or a total permission simply relieves people of responsibility altogether. We have not reached that position yet. Our situation is much more one of moral relativism and scepticism, like that denounced by Pascal in his *Pensées* ('*Plaisante justice qu'une rivière borne! Vérité au deça des Pyrénées, erreur au-delà'!* 'The travesty of justice bounded by a stream! Truth this side of the Pyrenees, error beyond!') Abortion permitted in Great Britain or in New York; abortion prohibited (that is practised illegally) in France or Italy. Disparities of this kind are no good to anyone; to the people of the different countries they seem terribly adventitious and arbitrary. I must now turn, therefore, to my second topic: the relation between legislation and personal life.

Legislation and personal life
Many maintain that the law should not interfere in this most private of all domains. It should be left entirely to the conscience of the couple concerned, the mother especially, assisted of course by the conscience of the medical specialist concerned, since abortion is still for the time being an operation requiring specialized medical assistance. The legislator would not need to know the motives or decisions either of the couple or of the doctor. There is an element of truth in this position.

It attaches great importance to the people most intimately concerned and does so without involving other more distant, more impersonal, and inevitably more technocratic official bodies. The introduction of judicial processes into this area brings with it attendant problems and dangers, since the law is almost invariably coloured by notions of punishment and repression. Since in most cases it would be a matter of intervening in situations which are already painful and traumatic in themselves, the result would only be to increase the stress of such situations by burdening it with the further tension of legal and judicial scrutiny.

Yet for at least two reasons this first position seems to me untenable. Is technical feasibility to be the only limiting factor in determining whether surgical intervention is permissible or not? To adopt this view would, it seems to me, involve a failure to distinguish between the different stages. For example, just as contraception is not the same thing as abortion, so foeticide is not at all comparable with infanticide. And surely it is the business of the law to reflect and reinforce these deep certitudes by legislation consistent with them. It is up to the law, therefore, to provide a framework. Without such a framework we should be helpless onlookers in situations where there was no legal safety barrier and only the conflict of opposing views. For some, everything would be forbidden and shameful; for others everything would be permissible and normal. Moreover, the purpose of the law is to provide a specific community with a reasonably convincing consensus so that the individual is not left entirely to his own devices, with all the strain and arbitrariness such isolation would entail. It would to my mind be an alarming prospect if parents and mothers, and doctors too, had to take sole ultimate responsibility on themselves with no formal indications as to what is desired, permitted, tolerated and authorised in the community to which they belong.

A statement of the law's attitude still seems to me quite indispensable, just as I also believe that absolute freedom of conscience too easily degenerates here into indifference. But the legal framework must not exclude the consideration of each case on its merits, and the power to authorise must also imply the power to refuse. But we also know that refusal can easily drive people to resort to illegal means, with all the hazards and inequalities this entails. Speaking as a moralist, I would not like us to take too jaundiced a view of legislative measures. After all, such measures simply underwrite the actual evolution of morals. Their aim is also to educate a community by means of correction and exhortation. Their chief objective should therefore be to promote serious discussion, to make people more aware of the issues and to help them, rather than to punish offences. A modern legal policy, like a modern health policy, should be preventive and global rather than merely curative and punitive.

Can we be more specific? What precisely is this moral consensus which, as I see it, would constitute a valid basis for legislation, accepting that such legislation would vary according to the different situations of different peoples? It could perhaps be stated as follows: Intervention in the interests of life is concerned primarily to protect the infant and to consider carefully the environment which is to receive it. Abortion will normally be a refusal of this protection and a failure on the part of this environment. In some cases however, failure to intervene may be a more irresponsible treatment of life than abortion itself. For such cases the law provides a frame of reference, entrusting to a commission which is representative of the relative consensus within a community, the responsibility for recommending, assisting, and also opposing an intervention, while at the same time avoiding any dramatisation of the situation by judicial procedures.

In my own country, France, we are faced with the need to draft new legislation to deal with those cases where abortion is to be permitted. Many proposals have been made as to the form this new legislation should take. The government, for example, has proposed a list of cases where a pregnant woman may ask for her pregnancy to be deliberately terminated: 'when the continuance of the pregnancy endangers her physical, mental or psychological health, either directly or because of long-term complications; the woman's age may constitute an aggravation of this danger; where there is a serious risk of congenital malformation or foetal deformity; where the pregnancy is the consequence of an assault or criminal act'. Centrist deputies add similar conditions: 'where the continuance of the pregnancy would clearly present the woman or possibly the family with a serious economic or psychological problem; the conditions required to permit a decision to terminate pregnancy in such cases will be set out in a formal statute'. The Communist group makes a very similar proposal: 'where the pregnancy presents the mother or the family with a social problem for which no immediate solution is available to them'. The combined group of Socialists and left-wing Radicals goes much further in the direction of a liberalisation of the law, stipulating simply that 'every woman can have an abortion on request in the first twelve weeks of her pregnancy'. 'If the pregnancy has gone beyond the twelfth week but has not reached the end of the twenty-fourth week, the woman, before requesting an abortion, must be interviewed by a doctor of her own choosing and by a family and social counsellor who will make their recommendation

on the advisability or otherwise of an abortion, giving the grounds for
their recommendation. The final decision rests with the woman herself.
If the pregnancy has gone beyond the twenty-fourth week, abortion is
permitted only if the continuance of the pregnancy endangers the
woman's life or if there is a risk of the child being born severely
handicapped.' Finally, the proposal of a United Socialist deputy: 'Every
woman can have an abortion, on request and without any age restriction, up to the end of the first twenty-four weeks of a pregnancy'.

This survey of proposals for legislation would be incomplete if we
omitted to mention the large group which is campaigning for the maintenance of existing French legislation which permits therapeutic abortion only in a very limited number of cases: 'if the use of medical
treatment which could lead to the termination of a pregnancy is required
in order to safeguard the mother's life when this is seriously endangered,
the doctor responsible for the treatment must without fail obtain the
opinion of two consultant physicians, one of whom must be selected
from the list of specialists attached to the Civil Tribunal; these con-
sultants must certify after examination and discussion that the life of
the mother can only be safeguarded by therapeutic treatment of this
kind'.

Under this existing legislation there were in France last year 162
legal abortions, hundreds of thousands of illegal abortions and, for
those people sufficiently well-informed, with the right connections and
money enough, a well-organized recourse to the facilities available in
neighbouring countries such as Switzerland, Holland and Great Britain,
where the abortion laws are more liberal. Despite this disturbing and
dangerous gap between the law and current morality, despite all the
psychological distress and social injustice of various kinds which it
entails, the group of those who are opposed to any proposals to
liberalize the legislation, even to the government's proposals, remains
a large and active one. Their object is to prevent any legalization of
what they consider to be murder, while on the other hand demanding
that society should provide the necessary help to ensure that every child
conceived will be welcomed by society and properly reared.

It seemed to me essential to describe in greater detail this painful,
emotion-laden and, I fear, deadlocked situation. On the one hand there
are those who wish to maintain the law as it stands, believing that it
serves as a dyke against any erosion of the principle of the sanctity of
life. There are others who are unwilling to wait for changes in legislation but wish to create here and now a situation where any prohibitions or penalties are regarded as intolerable, if they run counter to
the respect due to the wishes and desires of the mother as a person.

Between these two extremes there are all who would like to see the abortion laws liberalized to a substantial degree but not to the point of making abortion available simply on demand. They fear, mistakenly perhaps, that complete freedom of this kind would reduce abortion to the level of contraception; that it would equate abortion—which must always remain a matter of regret since it means terminating a living process already begun, even though there is no pressing temporal urgency—with contraception, which is a plan to prevent such a process from being initiated, with time on our side. In their view therefore, a liberal legal framework, which allows doctors to accede to the many requests for abortion, would fulfil the preventive and exhortative role we have seen belongs to the law, better than a legal framework which permitted complete freedom of abortion. They favour a form of legislation which would permit abortion in all cases where the unborn life represents a threat to the human person, but which at the same time would discourage repeated and irresponsible recourse to abortion, and encourage the use of contraception. This middle position is, of course, exposed to attacks from both sides, by those who consider such legislation as merely a hypocritical half-way house to complete permissiveness as well as by those who regard it as a determined campaign to defend legal prohibitions and medical embargoes.

At the time of writing it is impossible to forecast what action the French government will eventually take to reform our legislation. If it is too responsive to the conflicting demands of public opinion it will allow its action to be governed solely by its estimate of how the electorate will react, and will fail to provide a law capable of guiding society as a whole. In 1920, as we were emerging from the blood-letting of the First World War, we were given a law dictated by expediency, the aim of which was to increase the birth rate (which in fact it failed to do) and which outlawed not only abortion but even information on the subject of contraception. Are we now going to be given another such law, dictated by expediency, designed this time to fight the terrible scourge of clandestine abortions which results in the death of ten to a hundred times more people than die as a result of legal abortions? (Compared with at most only eight deaths in 100,000 abortion operations in the State of New York, the death rate among women illegally aborted in France today is a hundred in every hundred thousand!)

A law ceases to be merely opportunist legislation when it convinces people that it does in fact represent the right response today to a real situation; in other words, when a certain consensus emerges as to the best, or the least undesirable, of possible legislative solutions. For morality does not mean defending principles which are not practised, but helping people in distress and not failing to encourage them to take the necessary steps to ensure that such distress does not start all over again. To conclude this section I shall quote part of the explanation given for the proposals made by the government. This will help us to see clearly the conflict of values which is the context of this search for new legislation.

'Whenever the problem of abortion is raised, we encounter a serious conflict of opinion among the general public, as well as in religious, medical, and political circles, and even within the conscience of one and the same individual. If people even for a moment paused to consider the picture of one of these embryonic human beings killed after some weeks in the womb, how could anyone possibly proclaim the merits of abortion on demand as a way to individual or social liberation, and do so so loudly and calmly, as something entitling them to great respect and even as something to boast of? On the other hand, when we consider the whole ocean of misery endured by some women, how can we decide that abortion cannot be other than wrong, and regard such a decision as proof of our own moral superiority? Nor can all this uncertainty be cleared up by simply studying the legal provisions made in other countries. There too, the systems adopted range from the most repressive to the most permissive, with a wide variety of intermediate positions and a general tendency to move towards more liberal forms of legislation, although some countries where contraception was not widespread have had to modify their laws in the opposite direction in order to maintain their birth-rate.'

The abortion question thus makes a public issue of the twofold debate, that concerning the protection of life, the continuance of which, including the gradual and slow growth to personal existence, cannot be denied, and that concerning the protection of the human person when it finds itself threatened by a life which it has not desired and when the prospect of accepting this life is deeply distressing and even insupportable. Abortion is as old as mankind itself. What is new today is that it is becoming easier to practise it with the help of science and the permission of the law. I am convinced that the moral principle of the priority of the human person over life itself can here too guide the efforts of our legislators, even though, as we have seen, it is still not easy to devise a legislative framework which could make the termination of pregnancy a service of the human person yet not a cheapening of life itself.

The Judaeo-Christian tradition and abortion
It has become fashionable to blame the Judaeo-Christian tradition for turning abortion into a culpable and criminal act. Only in those countries

where this tradition has had and still has considerable influence does it prove difficult today to modify the feeling of radical revulsion associated with abortion. But the truth is that the situation is much more complex and confused. It is essential to try to disentangle the different elements, firstly in order to clarify the moral basis for new legislation in course of formulation, but secondly and above all, in order to discover if we can what the will of God is in this matter, in the conviction that this will represents what is best for man.

In ancient Greece the Hippocratic Oath undoubtedly included the condemnation of abortion ('I will not hand anyone poison if I am asked for it, nor will I put into any woman's hands the means to procure an abortion'). But this same Hippocrates gives certain prescriptions for abortion. The Greek philosophers accepted abortion both as a eugenic measure, to prevent the birth of deformed infants, and also as a means of keeping the increase in population in a city within reasonable bounds. Not only that; the exposure of new-born infants was much more commonly practised than was abortion. Aristotle writes: 'There should be a law concerning the future of new-born infants, to settle which of them should be exposed and which reared. It should not be lawful to rear any infant born deformed, that is deprived of some of their limbs. In a country where the abandonment of infants is illegal, in order to avoid the burden of over-population the maximum number of births should be decided and mothers aborted before the fruit of their womb has developed feeling and life, for it is here that we must distinguish between permissible suppression and that which is heinous' (*Politics* II:6). The idea that the foetus only subsequently acquired life (for male embryos after forty days, for female embryos after eighty days) would constitute the basis for this distinction between 'permissible' abortion and 'heinous' abortion throughout the entire period of medieval scholasticism. (Muslim canonists fixed the period as forty days, Christian canonists as 140 days.)

The Old Testament approach is completely different, for three obvious reasons. In the first place, far from being a question of eugenics, it is a matter of protecting the weak in the name of the merciful and compassionate Yahweh. In the second place, the concern to limit population growth simply did not arise since Israel always faced the threat of extermination, in captivity in Egypt as in exile in Babylon, and since Yahweh's blessing was always accompanied by the promise and the gift of a numerous posterity. Finally, the breath of life which comes from God is in the infant from the time of conception, long before its birth. It can even be said that the spirit of God is with the child even before conception, from the moment its birth is allowed and prophesied. Given these circumstances, it follows that we find no text in the Old

Testament authorising or excusing abortion. On the contrary, God's promise is of a time when no woman will ever willingly accept abortion: 'And ye shall serve the Lord your God . . . there shall nothing cast their young, nor be barren, in thy land: the number of thy days I will fulfil.' (*Exodus* 23:25-26). The only legal passages dealing with abortion concern the reparation to be made by anyone injuring a pregnant woman and causing her to miscarry and thus to lose her offspring (*Exodus* 21:22-25).

When the Hebraic tradition of the Old Testament came in contact with the ancient Graeco-Roman tradition, it produced several reactions. The Romans, Tacitus for example, were astonished that the Jews should be so naive politically as to prohibit infanticide which the Romans regarded as so essential to control population and to eliminate those whose unproductiveness made them a burden. That Christians did not attach the same theological importance to having children as the Jews had done is shown by the spiritual respect in which celibacy was held, by the warning to steer clear of genealogies (I *Timothy* 1:4 and *Titus* 3:9) and by the exhortations the apostles felt it necessary to address to Christian mothers encouraging them to persevere in maternity (I *Timothy* 2:15). Very early on, however, from the beginning of the second century, condemnations of abortion increased in frequency and would from then onwards be a characteristic feature of the Christian tradition in all its forms down to a very recent date.[1] Two motifs are inextricably interwoven here: firstly, a strictly Biblical and evangelical concern for the protection of the weak, the infant, the embryo, the gift of divine providence, against the policy of selection practised by the ancient world, which was accustomed to despise what it considered to be devoid of soul, value, beauty and autonomy. But there was another motif, derived from Pythagorean and Stoic philosophy, which was adopted and assimilated by the Christian tradition firstly at Alexandria and then in the synthesis developed by St. Augustine, namely the familiar idea of procreation as the natural goal of sexuality, with its corollary, branding everything running counter to this goal as unnatural, nature itself being identified with the intentions of God the Creator. Seneca wrote: 'A wise man should love his wife with discretion rather than with affection; he should control his impulses and not fling himself headlong into copulation. Nothing is more insane than to love a woman with the passion of an adulterer. Men should behave towards

---

[1] A detailed history of these condemnations is given in John Noonan (1965) *Contraception*, Harvard University Press.

their wives as husbands rather than as lovers' (Seneca *Fragments* 84, quoted by St. Jerome, *Contra Jovinianum* I, 49). It is clear from the context that this self-control will be shown by making procreation for the purposes of begetting children the goal of marriage, and by resisting the passions of love, equated now with concupiscence if this procreative purpose is deliberately evaded and rejected. This second motif carries us very far from the Biblical approach which views the passion of lovers as a supreme demonstration of the goodness of God's creation and as a parable of the divine covenant of election which binds God and His people Israel.

We are now sufficiently aware of this to realize just what is at stake in our present efforts to reinterpret the Bible and to reflect as Christians on this theme: how are we to keep to the evangelical insistence on the protection of the weak without perpetuating the infiltration of stoicism into Christian ethics by the view that any intervention must be regarded as unnatural, that is as deplorable and shameful, if it tries to forestall or prevent the procreative consequences of sexuality? For we must remember that the church fathers were just as severe in their condemnations of contraception, even in the makeshift and unreliable forms this took in their day, as they were in their condemnations of abortion, which was much more common, and of the custom of exposing unwanted new-born infants. It is clear from this that our situation today is very different from theirs, since we are in a position to distinguish scientifically and ethically between the three forms of intervention which they included in one and the same blanket condemnation. Here too, therefore, our problem is to sanctify the human person without making life itself sacrosanct.

As we saw at the beginning, what makes our thinking about abortion modern is the fact that it is inseparably bound up with advances in scientific knowledge with their two-edged consequences. There is certainly a difference, therefore, between today's question whether certain forms of abortion do not promote the quality of life and the question asked in earlier times whether or not it was permissible to suppress unwelcome lives by the practice of abortion. There remains, however, in the tradition deriving from the Bible, the fundamental requirement: respect and help your neighbour, especially when he is weak and defenceless! I realise that what I am to say as a Protestant theologian goes beyond what a Catholic theologian could probably say and still remain loyal to the declarations of his church's magisterium today. But if we believe now that the command of God does not impose a legalistic attitude to life itself and that there *are* cases where responsible love can with a good conscience help someone to have an abortion, it certainly does not follow from this that we regard it as essential to practice some such form of selection, a sort of obligatory eugenics, a rejection of life when it is attended with difficulties. For love does not eliminate difficulties; it helps us and others to bear them. This is a signpost to the road we should take. Not the way of a legalism which turns life's blessings into deadly inescapable necessities, nor the way of permissiveness which discovers reasons for evading rather than facing up to problems. Between these two dangers, of legalism on the one hand, and permissiveness on the other, there lies the way of solidarity which neither crushes the other nor leaves her to fend for herself alone, and which in some cases will assist her to find immediate liberation and in others to hope patiently for the future.

I conclude with a reminder that there are two ways in which the Judaeo-Christian tradition can become discredited: it can do so by saving its principles at the cost of shutting its eyes hypocritically to the facts; and it can do so by slavishly, if with a heavy heart and a bad conscience, following the direction in which morals are moving. But this Biblical tradition can be of help to human society if it bears witness to the God who gives succour and promise, the God who is personal freedom and not natural necessity, the God who is, and this above all perhaps, One who means life to be loved by man for man's sake, One who does not crush man under life's burden, just as Jesus insists that the Sabbath was made for man and not man for the Sabbath.

It is a most enriching experience for a theologian not to be left to himself and his own canons of truth when he reflects on so complex and urgent a problem as that of abortion. I am most grateful therefore for this opportunity of interdisciplinary and international discussion.

CHAPTER 11

Ethical issues in foetal diagnosis and abortion

Angelo Serra

Institute of Human Genetics,
Catholic University School of Medicine, Rome, Italy

Scientists, as well as governments and laymen, because of the rapid scientific and technological progress of the past decade, are dramatically faced with new, and until very recently, unpredictable, facets of old problems both in their scientific aspects and in their human and social implications. In the precise context of this consultation, old problems of the history of the evolution of the human species are re-emerging, with the profound difference that they now show the new mark of a hardly controllable 'man-steered evolution'. In fact the old forces of evolution, such as fertility, mutation, selection, migration and drift, which are still at work in human populations, are increasingly falling under the control of man's direct power.

The new, though conservative, man-controlled strategy has clearly been outlined by Neel (1970) and condensed in the following principles. First, stabilize the gene pool numerically. Second, protect the gene against damage. Third, improve the quality of life through parental choice based on genetic counselling and prenatal diagnosis. Fourth, improve the phenotypic expression of the individual genotype. The best means for the tactical development of this strategy should be those of eugenics, which 'are gradually becoming socially acceptable: birth control, therapeutic abortion and artificial insemination' (Crow 1972a).

It is obvious that man has the right, and at times the duty, to steer the evolution of its own species towards better physical, psychological and cultural levels. However, it is less obvious what a better level may be, and which are the best means to reach it. It is certainly true for instance, that 'In a world . . . increasingly concerned with the quality of human life, it will be taken for granted that children should be free from genetic disease' (WHO 1972). It is also obviously true that 'no one would argue for the preservation of physical and mental illness, or physical deformity or mental retardation' (Crow 1972a). But one may rightly question whether will it ever be possible to radically change the human germinal gene pool or make use of any means whatsoever, however disputable, to free humanity from suffering and misery. Two interrelated means of negative eugenics, one afforded by recent progress in cytogenetics and the other uncoveredly favoured by an apparently social consensus are foetal diagnosis and abortion. Their application obviously raises ethical issues. Precisely on these issues I shall submit a few statements for consideration and discussion, omitting all the strictly scientific and technical aspects which are already explained in other papers.

Foetal diagnosis

The recognition of genetic disorders of a human subject since its foetal stage is now made possible by the advanced techniques of amniocentesis, cytogenetics, microbiochemistry and, promisingly, foetoscopy. It is well known that abnormalities due to chromosomal aberrations and many metabolic disorders, originated by a deficiency or alteration of enzymes, can be diagnosed between the fifteenth and twentieth week of gestation. The present limitations of these techniques, the inherent risks for mother and foetus, and the necessary caution in the interpretation of the results are equally well known to every one who is engaged in the field, and have repeatedly been stressed in literature (Harris 1972; Epstein *et al.* 1972; Hilton *et al.* 1973). There is no doubt that in the next few years many technical improvements (Galjaard *et al.* 1972), and new diagnostic procedures, will allow for a greater number of early diagnosable disorders and for more rapid diagnosis.

The great potentialities of the prenatal diagnosis for a preventive medicine are obvious to all. Its application however raises ethical problems at three different levels. First at the level of the parents or the pregnant woman; second at the level of medical and/or genetic counsellor; third at the level of society.

The following principles could, in my opinion, afford a guide for their solution:

(1) The parents have the right to ask for a prenatal diagnosis if there are sufficient reasons to suspect that the prospective child has a considerable risk of being affected by some serious disorder detectable with the techniques in question. They have this right independently of any motivation which may underlie their request. The large diffusion, through mass media, of these new possibilities has really created in many women and parents a new psychological need, and consequently the right of knowing as much as they can of the health of their developing babies, just as they do for their newborn or growing up children.

As for any other disease, the pregnant woman or the parents will

not have, in general, a clear idea of the real risks of the foetus. Therefore, they shall ask the advice of a medical and/or genetic counsellor.

(2) The medical and/or genetic counsellor who is consulted for
a prenatal diagnosis, because of the above mentioned right of the
parents, has the duty to meet their request and, as much as possible,
their anxieties.

Firstly, he must decide whether there is a reasonable suspicion that
the prospective child is running a considerable risk of being affected
by some detectable serious disorder. This decision, however, may involve in practice many difficulties, of which the most important is that
only a small group of specialists can have the sufficient knowledge to
make the correct one. To obviate this difficulty I would agree with the
suggestion of Neel (1972)—though in a different perspective—of
creating a committee which periodically should update a list of those
defects that must be retained as detectable and the risks which
must be assumed as considerable. At present, the list should comprise, as a minimum, all the defects which are known to be correlated
with chromosomal aberrations, and about fifty metabolic disorders. The
risks which should be assumed as considerable for a prospective child
may be the following: (a) the 50 per cent risk for a male of being
affected by an X-linked recessive disease when the mother is the heterozygous carrier; (b) the 25 per cent risk of being affected by an autosomal recessive disorder when both parents are heterozygous carriers;
(c) the 1-15 per cent risk of being affected by a disorder due to an
unbalanced chromosomal complement, when one of the parents is a
balanced translocation carrier; (d) the 1.2-1.6 per cent risk of being
affected by a disorder due to a chromosomal aberration, when the
mother is more than thirty-five years old; (e) the 0.5-1 per cent risk
of being affected by a disorder due to a chromosomal aberration which
has already occurred in one sibling.

However, in deciding the extent of the degree of risk, one should
also reflect upon the seriousness of the suspected disorder, and the
possibility of curing it.

Secondly, the medical counsellor must fully and intelligibly explain
to the counselee: (a) the risks to the mother and to the foetus from
amniocentesis; (b) the risks of unsuccessful and/or incorrect analysis;
(c) the precise inferences to be drawn concerning the health of the
prospective child from a negative result.

Only if all these arguments are thoroughly discussed with the interested
parents or woman, can they then make an intelligent and moral decision,
with full responsibility, about whether or not to undertake the analysis
with all the possible consequences.

Thirdly, no pressure of any kind must be put by the counsellor on the parents or the woman about their action upon the foetus, when the results of the analysis will be known. I feel that this is the most delicate and critical point. In the current scientific literature on the subject there are clear statements: 'It is imperative that . . . before amniocentesis . . . a firm decision is made to interrupt the pregnancy, if the suspected disorder is proved by the amniotic fluid examination' (Fuchs 1972a). 'In practice, the decision about termination would almost always have been made earlier, since amniocentesis would not have been undertaken at all unless termination were legal and parents had agreed that they would want termination if a condition were found which would seriously handicap the child' (Carter 1972). 'I still feel that if parents frankly say: "we are going to keep this pregnancy regardless", it is wrong to undertake amniocentesis' (Macintyre 1972a). 'In my opinion intra-uterine diagnosis should be offered to those families at risk who, having understood the issues, are prepared in the light of their own personal, social, economic, religious and ethical circumstances to consider selective abortion' (Fraser 1972a).

I think that conditioning the prenatal diagnosis to a previous decision of aborting an abnormal foetus is equivalent to unjustly denying a due analysis and imposing a line of action which constrains the freedom of the counselee. In fact, the duty of the counsellor extends as much as the right of the counselee. As regards the point in question, the right of the counselee in relation to the counsellor is the right to have a prenatal diagnosis. The rights of the counselee relative to the foetus derive, on the contrary, from the relation parents-foetus and are, therefore, absolutely outside the relation counselee-counsellor. Moreover I assume it as fundamental that no counsellor force his own personal views upon the counselee. By analogy, though well aware of the differences, one has the right to know if he wants to, whether he is affected by cancer; and the corresponding duty of the doctor is to tell him what he wants. But the decision whether to undertake a chirurgical treatment or not is entirely outside the field of the established relation patient-doctor.

Finally, the medical counsellor must be sensible to the psychological conflicts of the counselees. It is to be underlined that the anxiety of many couples about the health of the foetus is in fact highly exaggerated by the anxiety of what they shall do when they know the answer. This is a common experience, but Fletcher (1972) has recently given a clear evidence of this psychological background through an analysis of twenty-five couples who underwent amniocentesis for pre-natal diagnosis, of which there were eleven Protestant, four Hebrew, two Catholic, five of mixed religion, and three with no religious affiliation. Though personally admitting that 'the interest of preservation of the family bond and its resources may, in specific cases, be chosen above the interest of preserving until birth the life of a severely deformed infant for whom no treatment is available' he, however, stresses the fact that the studied couples 'all show signs of moral suffering', and explains that 'moral suffering occurs when highly motivated parents who desire children intensely, even desperately, are caught between the rightness of protecting their families from the great strains which genetic disease may place upon them and the rightness of unconditional caring for the life of their conceived child'.

This psychologically conflicting situation is, by itself, a strong argument against placing any further extrinsic pressure upon the couple who have to make their decision with absolute autonomy. Evidently, the condition ordinarily requested for amniocentesis, as mentioned above, places such a pressure upon the couple. On the other side, this psychological state of the counselees urges a special attention from the counsellor, and, possibly, the intervention of trained psychologists, in order to help the couples in the solution of their conflicts. In this respect, the knowledge of the real condition of the foetus may favour the solution in the greatest number of cases.

(3) Society has the duty to provide the means for prenatal diagnosis to every one who has the right to ask for it. This duty originates from the right that, in the circumstances which were discussed above, the individuals of the community have to ask for this analysis, and it is part of the general obligation of the society to promote the health of the community. Indeed, even within the limits defined in a preceding section and disregarding the possibility of prenatal treatments in the near future, foetal diagnosis, while responding to a new general demand, could function as a highly sensitive monitoring system, able to locate subjects and families in need of special and, in certain instances, preventive care.

The problem of the cost, which represents a burden to society, is secondary to this obligation. No matter what the cost may be, an intelligent plan to be gradually developed, both in its scientific and practical aspects, will certainly give man a new power for mastering genetic disease.

Abortion

Pregnancy termination for several different purposes, as birth control, family economical and psychological well-being, and, very recently, eugenics, is increasingly socially accepted, widely practised and legally protected.

Eugenic, or otherwise therapeutic, abortion is advocated as the final act of a positive prenatal diagnosis. 'If such an analysis clearly indicates the presence of a hereditary disease, the foetus can be aborted' (Freese 1972). 'The only currently possible solution . . . is restricted to termination of particular pregnancies by therapeutic abortion . . . Our currently changing attitudes about practising negative eugenics, by means of intelligent selection for therapeutic abortion, must be encouraged' (Hirschhorn 1972). 'When a diagnosis of a serious genetic disorder has been made by amniocentesis, the pregnancy should be terminated without delay' (Fuchs 1972a).

The support to this plea is of double order: scientific and humanitarian. 'Scientifically, this kind of eugenics is by far the most desirable approach to hereditary disease, because it avoids human misery and also somewhat reduces the frequency of defective genetic information in the gene pool' (Freese 1972). 'The enormous potential of these methods, in combination with selective abortion, for reducing the toll of serious genetic disease is obvious' (Miller 1972). 'The humanitarian gains from such abortions are enormous' (Crow 1972). 'I find it difficult to see in our recent and continuing reproductive performance, condemning so many infants to a miserable death and so many of the survivors to marginal diets incompatible with full physical and mental development, any greater respect for the quality of human existence than evidenced by our primitive ancestors', who seem 'to have recognized the need for curbing reproduction, and when the limited means at disposal for so doing failed then practised infanticide, especially directed towards the defective' (Neel 1972). 'In order to prevent the birth of a terribly defective child, and the emotional and economic destruction of a family unit, therapeutic abortion is the better of two unhappy choices' (Macintyre 1972b).

These are only a few of the authoritative quotations of an impressive literature on the subject. Such a general consensus among scientists, that in many countries is upheld by the law, would seem implicitly to show that ethical and social problems connected with a direct and deliberate abortion either do not exist, or are negligible, or are already solved. My impression is that no one fails to recognize that those problems really exist, and are not trivial; but, because of the difficulties met with in harmonizing conflicting values, one is tempted to skip them over and rather accept the more common attitude of the environmental culture and act accordingly. Crow (1972b) explicitly points out: 'Actually, public acceptance of abortion as a means of birth limitation and as a right of the individual pregnant woman is now so widespread that a discussion of reservations about therapeutic abortion seems almost anachronistic'.

While experiencing these difficulties myself, I shall propose a few ideas that I assume as fundamental for the correct solution of the ethical problems involved in the abortion of a foetus diagnosed as genetically defective.

The foetus, at the time when the diagnosis can be made, is already a human being. I think that no one who has the rudiments of genetics and human embryology can deny this. However it has recently been objected (Beirnaert 1970; Antoine 1971; Ribes 1973) that 'human being' is not equivalent to 'man', and stated that a 'human being' becomes a 'man' only if it is 'humanized'. The necessary and sufficient condition for the 'humanization' of a 'human foetus' would essentially be that the foetus be recognized and/or accepted by parents and/or society as a member of the family and/or community.

This would seem the less arbitrary criterion to solve the central point of all discussion, namely 'at what stage in pregnancy does the foetus enter the fraternity of man, so that terminating its existence raises the same ethical problem as terminating the existence of any other human being?' (Neel 1972). But actually it is not, since this criterion calls for another more vital point: when and for what reasons do parents and society have the right or the duty of rejecting a living human foetus, if they have this right or duty at all?

Therefore, one must consider from one side the rights of the foetus and from the other the rights and duties of parents and society.

The intrinsic right of a human foetus is the right to its own appropriate development, not to its health. Precisely as the right of each individual is to have all that is necessary to preserve or recover its health, not the health itself. It is an unfortunate but real fact that disease is an integrating and inescapable part of human life, for every human being.

This essential right cannot be lost by the foetus, whatever may be the chromosomal or gene abnormality or genetic disorder it carries. No human being can lose its right to life because its health is seriously physically and/or mentally compromised. If one admits the contrary at an initial point whatsover of the growth curve of a subject then he should also admit that the same right may be lost at any other point along the life curve. Indeed, the humanitarian motive, which is ordinarily invoked as justification for terminating the life of a foetus, has equal validity for any human being at any time when the physical and/or mental health are gravely impaired.

It is also clear, from the other side, that the acquired certainty that the prospective child will be affected by a serious genetic disorder somehow modifies the attitude of parents towards the foetus. The knowledge, or the accumulated experience that parents have of a previously affected child, forces them to believe that such a type of life may be so terribly miserable that death before birth is preferable. The great amount of resources for the care of an unhealthy child, and the continuous psychological stress to themselves and to other children, make them feel that the addition of a new potentially abnormal child would be an unpleasant and oppressive load which they can and must not bear. They may be emotionally so involved as to feel that they have the right of terminating a pregnancy.

Although such circumstances can frequently occur, one however can hardly find convincing arguments for asserting that the will to avoid suffering for a prospective child and the right of parents and children to a better life, can give them the right to terminate another human life, even though it is miserable in our eyes. On the contrary, the respect for the whole human life, from its beginning to its end, seems to be a duty so important and of such consequences that any presumed right against life must be evidently proved.

This applies also to society. Indeed, the right of society to provide for the genetic health of the present and future generations must be balanced by its duty to protect the life of each human subject of the community. Elementary genetic considerations, and a little more sophisticated elaboration (Motulsky *et al.* 1971; Neel 1972; Fraser 1972*a*, 1972*b*), show the claim that selective abortion represents the best scientific means to free our genetic pool from deleterious information, is at least a naïve one or rather fallacious. At the population level, genetically beneficial effects from selective abortion could be achieved for dominant lethal and sub-lethal genes, and for chromosomal aberrations without translocation heterozygotes. In these cases, assuming that the application of prenatal diagnosis could be extended to the entire population, defective genes and chromosomes would actually be eliminated in each generation. But with respect to autosomal and X-linked recessive genes, and chromosomal aberrations with balanced translocation carriers, because of reproductive compensation, which increases the relative number of heterozygotes, the frequency of deleterious genes and chromosomes would tend, generation after generation, to a new higher equilibrium. Therefore in these cases selective abortion would really have long-term dysgenic effects, though small and perceptible after a time span of many generations, except for resorting to the absolutely unhuman strategy of also aborting the heterozygotes.

It is difficult to understand how such theoretical conclusions, which should have suggested some hesitation in the defence of selective abortion for eugenic reasons, have, to the contrary, stimulated opinions like these: 'I think it is a very pertinent question whether we should not try to get rid of heterozygotes as well as homozygotes . . . There is no reason why we cannot continue the approach, using the same technique of amniocentesis and selective interruption of pregnancy on the daughters if they turn out to be carriers, and continue that for generation after generation' (Fuchs 1972b). 'In the future, we should also discuss the role of the heterozygous carrier. For example, if one aborts a male foetus with muscular dystrophy or haemophilia, is one justified in permitting a female foetus, who is a known carrier of these same defects, to come to term so that the problem of diagnosis will repeat itself in the next generation?' (Hsia 1972). 'I would particularly agree with the case of a translocation, because here you are not really aborting an essentially normal infant, but one who is going to have a high risk of having abnormal offspring himself' (Hirschhorn 1972b). 'I don't think we should overwhelmingly be concerned about aborting a normal foetus. For social reason this is going to be done more and more commonly' (Littlefield 1972).

Disregarding this possibility as something evidently unhuman, the overall effect of selective abortion, applied to all foetuses homozygous for deleterious genes or carriers of abnormal chromosomes, would then be that of reducing the number of genetically defective individuals in one generation.

Certainly the economic advantage for society, alleviated of the burden of their care, may be considerable. But one may rightly ask: in order to lower the number of seriously handicapped human subjects and restrain the expenses for their care, has society the right to condemn them to death? Has not society rather the duty to make any effort, firstly, to educate people, through intelligently used mass media and genetic counselling services, to a controlled fertility, and, secondly, to stimulate a greater advancement in the therapy of genetic disease? This seems to me the only way society has to accomplish both, its duty to protect human life and its right to provide for the genetic health of the community. True, it will require time to create this sense of respect for life and responsibility in reproduction. During this time genetically defective individuals will still represent a good portion of unhealthy people. But the long-term effect of this policy, where the respect for life equals the responsibility in reproduction, will likely be a better humanity in which man may more humanly and rationally guide his own evolution.

References

ANTOINE, P. (1971) Nâitre à une vie d'homme. *Cahiers Laennec Mars.* **23**.

BEIRNAERT, L. (1970) L'avortement est-il un infanticide? *Etudes.* Nov. **520**.

CARTER, C. O. (1972) Practical aspects of early diagnosis. *In* Harris, Maureen (ed.). See below, p. 18.

CROW, J. F. (1972*a*) The dilemma of nearly neutral mutations: how important are they for evolution and human welfare? *Journal of Heredity.* **63**, 306.

—(1972*b*) (Introductory remark.) *In* Bergsma, D. (ed.) Advances in human genetics and their impact in society. *Birth Defects: Original Article Series.* **8**, 5.

EPSTEIN, Ch. J., SCHNEIDER, E. L., CONTE, F. A. & FRIEDMAN, S. (1972). Prenatal detection of genetic disorders. *Annals of Human Genetics.* **24**, 214.

FLETCHER, J. (1972) The brink: the parent-child bond in the genetic revolution. *Theological Studies.* **33**, 457.

FRASER, G. R. (1972*a*) Genetical implications of antenatal diagnosis. *Bulletin of the European Society of Human Genetics.* No. 98. (Reproduced in *Annales de Genetique.* 1973 **16**, 5.)

—(1972*b*) Selective abortion, gametic selection and the X chromosome. *American Journal of Human Genetics.* **24**, 359.

FREESE, E. (1972) (ed.) *The Prospects of Gene Therapy.* Fogarty International Center Publication Report. DHEW Pub. No. (NIH) 72-61. p. 2.

FUCHS, F. (1972*a*) Amniocentesis: techniques and complications. *In* Harris, Maureen (ed.). See below, p. 11.

—(1972*b*) Discussion to the paper of Hsia, D.Y.Y. See below, p. 125.

GALJAARD, H., FERNANDES, J., JAHODOVA, M., KOSTER, J. F. & NIERMEIJER, M. F. (1972) Prenatal diagnosis of genetic disease. *Bulletin of the European Society of Human Genetics.* Nov. **79**.

HARRIS, Maureen (ed.) (1972) *Ethical Problems in Human Genetics: Early Diagnosis of Genetic Defects.* Fogarty International Center Publication Proceedings No. 6, DHEW Pub. No. (NIH) (National Technical Information Service, US Dept. of Commerce.)

HILTON, B., CALLAHAN, D., HARRIS, Maureen, CONDLIFFE, P. & BERKLEY, B. (eds.) (1973) *Ethical Issues in Human Genetics: Genetic Counseling and the Use of Genetic Knowledge.* Fogarty International Center Publication Proceedings No. 13. (Plenum Publishing Corp.: New York.)

HIRSCHHORN, K. (1972*a*) Discussion to the paper of Lubs, H. A. See below.

—(1972*b*) Practical and ethical problems in human genetics. *Birth Defects: Original Article Series.* **8**, 17.

HSIA, D. Y. Y. (1972) Detection of heterozygotes. *In* Harris, Maureen (ed.). See above. p. 105.

LITTLEFIELD, J. W. (1972) Discussion to the paper of Lubs, H. A. See below. p. 85.

LUBS, H. A. (1972) Cytogenic problems in antenatal diagnosis. *In* Harris, Maureen (ed.). See above. p. 67.

MACINTYRE, M. N. (1972*a*) Discussion to the paper of Nadler, H. See below. p. 143.

—(1972*b*) Professional responsibility in prenatal genetic evaluation. *Birth Defects: Original Article Series.* **8**, 31.

MILLER, O. J. (1972) An overview of problems arising from amniocentesis. *In* Harris, Maureen (ed.). See above. p. 23.

MOTULSKY, A. G., FRASER, G. R. & FELSENSTEIN, J. (1971) Public health and long-term genetic implications of intrauterine diagnosis and selective abortion. *Birth Defects: Original Article Series*. **7**, 22.

NADLER, H. L. (1972) Risks in amniocentesis *In* Harris, Maureen (ed.). See above p. 129.

NEEL, J. V. (1970) Lessons from a 'primitive' people. *Science*. **170**, 815.
—(1972) Ethical issues resulting from prenatal diagnosis. *In* Harris, Maureen (ed.) See above. p. 219.

RIBES, B. (1973) Pour une reforme de la législation française relative a l'avortement. *Etudes*. Jan. 66.

WORLD HEALTH ORGANIZATION. (1972) Genetic disorders: prevention, treatment and rehabilitation. *WHO Technical Report*. Series No. **497**, 5.

CHAPTER 12

Legal issues in foetal diagnosis and abortion

Alexander Morgan Capron

University of Pennsylvania Law School, Philadelphia, USA

It is best to begin with a statement of the limitations of what follows. I address the topic of prenatal diagnosis and abortion as a lawyer trained in a common law system; we will have to rely on the comments of those versed in the comparative law of the code-based European legal systems to suggest issues which do not emerge from my analysis. I have attempted to address the *legal issues* raised by prenatal diagnosis and abortion rather than to state *the law* on these subjects (not in the least because there is little law directly on the point). Yet 'legal issues' are not immutable but are shaped as much by the legal orientation of the person who perceives them as his statement of the law would be. In reviewing both the 'public law' and 'private law' issues, I am influenced by a document which is fairly unique in the common law world, the Constitution of the United States. As you are probably already aware, that document—which is of such great importance in large areas of American jurisprudence—has special relevance today on the subject of abortion, about which our Supreme Court has recently had some far-reaching things to say. While these factors may be said to constrict my comments—within the compass of the American common law—other factors may tend to broaden them, for I shall address myself to issues which go beyond those raised in law suits and employ an analysis which looks at the roles played by the various participants in decision-making and attempts to ask 'what should the law be?'.

Foetal diagnosis and abortion: a necessary connection?
The conjunction of 'foetal diagnosis' and 'abortion' in the topic assigned me suggests that the planners of this consultation on genetics may have had in mind that the two are tied together in practice. Before moving on to the heart of the topic, we must ask whether this indeed is, or ought to be, the case.

There are indications in the literature that many (perhaps most) people involved in medical genetics regard abortion to be linked with prenatal diagnosis. For example, one physician recently wrote: 'It also is imperative that the parents make a decision regarding termination of the pregnancy if a chromosome abnormality is found, prior to the date of amniocentesis. Otherwise, there is no valid reason for performing this procedure' (Jones 1972).

Such a medical policy has two effects. First, it means that, at present, knowledge about genetically-caused conditions is only available to those prospective parents who agree in advance to abort an affected foetus, while those who are uncertain about abortion, or who desire information so as to prepare themselves for the birth of an affected infant, are denied this medical procedure. Second, the willingness of the physician to undertake the prenatal diagnosis demonstrates that he regards the condition for which the screening has been undertaken to be grave enough to justify abortion of the foetus.

This state of affairs is regrettable, because it clouds what ought to be the separate analysis of the merits of the two procedures, foetal diagnosis and abortion, and because it imposes what seem to me to be improper restrictions on the medical procedures involved.

I have taken the practice to be that foetal diagnosis is conditioned upon an agreement to abort. If it appeared that abortion were restricted to those cases in which a foetus had been diagnosed as defective, another set of objections could be raised. I do not believe that such a diagnosis is anywhere taken to be the sole (or even primary) grounds for abortion, and the debate over abortion goes on largely without reference to such genetic issues. Both issues of foetal diagnosis and abortion are illustrated if one examines the two justifications which would probably be given by physicians for restricting amniocentesis to those cases in which an abortion is agreed to ahead of time. Firstly it might be said that the capability to perform amniocentesis is a 'scarce resource' which may properly be limited to those cases in which the resulting diagnosis will 'be put to use' or 'will do some good'. Secondly, it might be argued that the procedure involves some appreciable risk to mother and foetus and that such risk is unjustified where there is no intention to abort an affected foetus. The latter argument strikes me as one which relates to the merits of the procedure—that is, whether amniocentesis is 'safe' (in terms of morbidity/mortality for pregnant woman, potential for injury or death of unaffected foetus, and so on), and how its risk compares with the risk of bearing a child with the condition being screened for. Of course, the decision whether to undertake amniocentesis will depend in each individual case upon the parents' view of the harm which would be caused by the birth of an affected child (in the absence of screenings) and this is plainly a judgment which goes beyond medical expertise. But, at least, this justification for restricting amniocentesis begins with an initial 'medical' issue. By contrast, the first justification is utterly and entirely a value judgment. Yet, as so often turns out to be the case when a careful analysis is made of medical practice, the decision has been framed in such a way as to appear to be a 'medical' judgment that ought properly be made by the physicians.

Law: mediator of conflicting interests

As this preliminary discussion has already suggested, the legal analysis quickly leads one to ask: what are the conflicting interests and by whom are they to be formulated and resolved? For our purposes, I have identified four sets of participants who have definable interests and who may play some role in decision-making about alternatives that effect those interests. They are: (1) physician-investigators, (2) parents and (3) children (who together might be termed 'patients'), and (4) collective bodies, such as the professions and the state.

By 'the state' I mean any organ of government, and not solely (in American terms) *state* rather than *federal* government. For a fuller and somewhat different exploration of the role of the various participants in decision-making, *see* Capron (1972). The role of the law in this model, then, is to mediate the conflicts and to provide a means of minimizing the harm that these conflicts may cause. Let us look at each in turn.

Individual v. individual

There are two major conflicts of individual interests: physician-investigators' interests versus those of patients', and parents' interests versus those of their progeny. In ordinary medical practice, the interests of the physician are assumed to be congruent with those of the patient; the 'ethical physician' is supposed to act only in his patient's 'best interests'. As is increasingly noted, particularly by sociologists and ethicists, there are serious problems with this assumption, since the values of the physician may not coincide with those of the patient; indeed, there is good reason to believe that the personality type of physicians and the training they receive inculcates them with many values not generally shared in society. Often, as was illustrated by the discussion of the medical practice of linking abortion to prenatal diagnosis, the divergence of values goes unnoticed because 'value judgments' are consciously or unconsciously disguised as medical decisions which physicians alone are competent to make without input from their patients.

Amniocentesis is not, however, ordinary medicine, and the physician acts not solely as therapist but also as investigator, with an interest in the scientific knowledge which may be gained through the application of this new technique to clinical cases.

To state that a medical procedure is 'experimental' is not, of course, to condemn it. Indeed, in recent years Western culture has been deeply committed to the notion that medicine will 'progress' and give man ever greater powers over disease and distress. Yet the law does recognize that medical innovation demands special scrutiny lest the potential conflicts of interests between physician-investigator and patient-subject go unrecognized and uncontrolled. The locus of authority here resides with our first two participants: physician and patient, and primary reliance has been placed on making sure that the patient has given his or her 'voluntary, informed consent', a concept developed in cases involving therapeutic interventions[1] but now applied to experimental ones as well (US DHEW 1971). The professions and the state have also become involved in the process, initially through the promulgation of ethical standards, such as the *Nuremberg Code* and the *Declaration of Helsinki*, and more recently through the requirement that all research sponsored by the Federal government must first be reviewed by an institutional committee concerned with protecting the human subjects from harm. In addition to informed consent, such codes and committees are concerned with limiting the risks to which subjects are exposed (by assuring that the experiment is well-designed and has been preceded by the necessary trials in animals), that the investigators are properly qualified to undertake the research, and that the research will yield benefits (to subjects, society or science) which exceed the harm they may create. Obviously, this listing of the considerations which are raised by medical experimentation merely suggests questions and does not answer them—nor could I hope to do so in this limited format. Suffice it to say that amniocentesis and the other means of prenatal diagnosis remain at the moment experimental techniques with uncertain risks and benefits.

The experimental nature of prenatal diagnosis raises similar issues for the foetus as patient as it does for the pregnant woman, but there is an additional aspect in the case of the foetus which leads to the question of the second conflict between individual interests mentioned at the outset of this section: the potential divergence of parental interest versus the interest of the foetus. Since the foetus is incapable of giving

---

[1] *See, e.g., Cobbs* v. *Grant,* 502 P. 2d 1 (Cal. 1972); *Natanson* v. *Kline,* 186 Kan. 393, 350 P. 2d 1093 (1960).

'informed consent' for himself, that responsibility is given by law to his parents. Even though the procedure involved may be experimental, the parents' authority to consent would not usually be doubted, provided that the procedure is intended at least in part to benefit the foetus. Yet in the present situation, this may not be the case, depending upon the purpose for which amniocentesis is undertaken. This points up the question: who or what is being treated? If the diagnosis will be used to improve delivery or prenatal care, then the foetus is the patient; if the diagnosis is intended to prepare the parents for the eventuality of a child with genetic or chromosomal disorder, then the parents seem to be the patients; and if diagnosis is intended to lead to 'therapeutic abortion' of an affected foetus, then the patient may be society, the family, or perhaps the foetus.

The latter possibility—that the foetus should be considered the patient here, that is, a subject of physicians' desire to help rather than merely the object of their desire to remove 'malignant' growths—is sharply disputed by those who find this use of the word 'therapy' an abomination. Ramsey (1972), for example, argues that it is ridiculous to construe treatment 'to include killing the patient for his own sake in order that he may not have a life deemed by others not to be worth living'.

Arguments of this sort are reflected in a group of recent cases based on what some have termed an attempt to recover for 'wrongful life' (Tedeschi 1966). In the leading case, *Gleitman* v. *Cosgrove*,[2] the New Jersey Supreme Court held that neither parents nor child had an actionable claim against a physician who erroneously advised a woman that the german measles she suffered during the first month of pregnancy 'would have no effect at all on her child'.[3] The physician knew the risk of rubella damage to be about 25 per cent, but he withheld this information because he believed it unfair to abort three healthy foetuses to avoid one diseased one. Although the justices assumed that the mother could legally have obtained an abortion, they ruled that the parents could not recover because an abortion would have violated 'the preciousness of human life' and that the child was foreclosed because he would 'not have been born at all' had his parents carried out the abortion.

The New Jersey court's position is somewhat narrower than Professor Ramsey's, but it comes down to the same point. Apparently, the court believed that life with any handicap is *per se* better than no life at all:

---

[2] 49 N.J. 22, 227 A.2d 689 (1967). *See also Williams* v. *New York,* 18 N.Y. 2d 481, 223 N.E. 2d 343 (1966); *Zepeda* v. *Zepeda,* 41 Ill. App. 2d 240, 190 N.E. 2d 849 (1963), *cert. denied,* 379 U.S. 945 (1964).
[3] 49 N.J. at 24, 227 A.2d at 690.

the child could not sue the physician 'for his life', although it was heavily burdened with the rubella-caused injuries, because without his life he would not be able to sue at all. But, Professor Ramsey notwithstanding, it does not seem to me ridiculous or even reprehensible to say that in certain circumstances life may be 'a fate worse than death', and that society may find it acceptable to allow the prospective parents to make this choice for their damaged foetus. Indeed, the central error in the *Gleitman* decision is in the framing of the injury as being for 'wrongful life'. The wrong actually perpetrated by the physician was in keeping necessary information from the parents, who had the right to make the decision, and instead arrogating the decision to himself (Capron 1973).

Individual v. group

A further issue which is raised by the quotation from Professor Ramsey is whether, in discussing foetal diagnosis and abortion, one is talking about a patient who is a 'person' in the usual sense of the word. In its decisions earlier this year,[4] which effectively struck down the anti-abortion statutes then existing in most states, the United States Supreme Court addressed the issue in just these terms. On the one hand, the Court found a constitutionally-based 'right to privacy' which 'is broad enough to encompass a woman's decision whether or not to terminate her pregnancy',[5] while on the other hand the developing foetus is not a 'person', in constitutional terms, though it has substantial rights after viability (*circa* twenty-four weeks). Although the conflict here is one between the interests of the parents and those of the foetus, the abortion decision provides an example of individual versus group conflict because of the active part played in decision-making by the state. The reason for this is obvious: although the conflict involves the rights of individuals, one of them (namely the foetus) is unable to express its wishes and powerless to enforce them. Thus, the state substituted its judgment for that of the foetus, by erecting an absolute (or near absolute) ban on abortions. The absolute nature of the prohibition was attempted to be justified on the basis that the object of its concern—the foetus— deserved the same protection against 'murder' accorded to other 'persons'. Once the basis of the analogy is questioned, as the Court did, the propriety of the ban on abortions is cast into doubt. As a matter of logic, however, the opposite result (namely the one reached in *Roe* v. *Wade* that the mother's rights must predominate) is far from ineluctable: there are many other ways in which the 'rights' of a person may

[4] *Roe* v. *Wade*, 410 U.S. 113 (1973); *Doe* v. *Bolton*, 410 U.S. 179 (1973).
[5] 410 U.S. at 153.

be curtailed, even severely, to benefit or protect non-persons.

In addition to demonstrating society's collective interest in the protection of the foetus from the adverse interest of the mother, the anti-abortion statutes also reflected what was regarded as society's own interest in 'public decency' although many commentators are critical of laws designed to dictate 'morality' (Hart 1961; Devlin 1965). Interestingly, there is another aspect of the abortion controversy in which it appears that society's collective interest may be adverse to that of the *foetus* rather than that of the mother. 'Modern' abortion statues typically permit abortion when there is a substantial risk that the child will be born with 'grave physical or mental defects'.[6] This reflects, it seems to me, not only a realization (as was suggested in the preceding subsection) that in the exercise of substituted judgment one might conclude that the foetus would 'rather not be born'; it also shows a concern on the part of the state to conserve medical resources. I can see no other conclusion from the state's permitting the abortion of certain foetuses who will probably place a heavy demand on our collective resources if they are born with serious disease or deformity, at the same time that abortion is prohibited in most instances where such 'reasons' are absent.

A concern for the conservation of funds and medical resources is a perfectly legitimate, even laudable, collective concern. The invocation of this concern in the context of prenatal diagnosis and abortion, for 'genetic reasons' however, is sure to raise some very ticklish problems. An example of the crosscurrents at play here may be useful. At present, neonatal screening for phenylketonuria (PKU) (and in some states, other inborn errors of metabolism as well) is mandated by statute in forty-three American jurisdictions. The justification given for this invasion of the 'privacy' of the baby and its parents is that mental retardation may be avoided if a child with PKU is promptly detected and placed on a diet low in phenylalanine. The state in most instances has to support the PKU retardate for life; such institutional care for one PKU child is said to be more costly than screening 18,000 newborns and treating the one affected child. Although the economics involved is probably very faulty (because it leaves out many of the intangible or difficult-to-calculate costs of treating an affected child), such considerations seem entirely proper for state legislatures and executives to consider in drawing up and applying laws. If a method were available to detect PKU prenatally rather than postnatally, however, would it be equally proper for the state to conclude that amniocentesis should be performed in all pregnancies 'at risk' for PKU, with abortion to follow if a PKU baby were detected, since the cost of these prenatal

[6] *See, e.g.,* American Law Institute, *Model Penal Code* §230.3.

procedures are much less than postnatal testing and treatment?

An additional matter, which deserves to be mentioned again though it need not be discussed at length, is the tendency of society to delegate group decisions to experts. This is particularly true in the abortion area; in the abortion cases, the court left the decision to abort up to the mother with the understanding that 'abuses' would be prevented by the exercise of 'medical judgment'.

Present v. future

There is no need for me to rehearse the debate concerning the dangers, or lack thereof, to the future of the human species if the gene pool is not protected against medicine's demonstrated propensity to keep the 'unfit' alive and allow them to procreate. The question I would like to pose is: how adept is society (through the law) at mediating the conflict between present and future interests?

The practical and theoretical problems suggested in the foregoing discussion of group interests are, if anything, sure to be magnified rather than reduced when society is attempting to determine what *will be* beneficial genetically in the future rather than what *is* beneficial now. A limitation on present conduct (for example, reproductive behaviour) based on a desire to improve the genetic heritage of future generations is dependent upon a clear understanding not only of what is collectively desirable but also of what the general environment of the future will be like, particularly in the medical sphere. The current wave of concern for the preservation of the environment thus provides at best a strained analogy. It is likely—although far from irrefutable—that future generations will be better off if we restrain our present mad consumption of natural resources; but it is difficult to be sure exactly what 'conservation' is in the genetic area—especially since man is not only an *actor* in the process of change but also an *object* of the evolutionary process as well.

I am assuming that the limitations placed on present choices intended to benefit the future are collectively decided upon (for example, by the government). Purely individual decision-making would raise fewer problems, primarily because individual decisions tend to cancel each other out and there would be less chance of setting the whole gene pool off in a bad direction. Of course, if the 'choices' of individuals are in actuality decisions dictated by physicians or other professional geneticists, the danger of what may be irrevocable harm would again loom large. Moreover, allowing geneticists to make these decisions would represent an improper arrogation of authority to them to impose their value preferences about the desirable future society under the guise of 'professional judgment'.

If it is likely that any 'future-oriented' limitations would therefore have to be formulated and imposed by the state, we must inquire whether such limitations would impose an impermissible restraint on individual choice. (Here, again, my comments perforce take on a distinctly American cast.) More than thirty years ago, in holding unconstitional a statute permitting the sterilization of 'habitual criminals', the Supreme Court declared that the legislation touched on 'one of the basic civil rights of man. Marriage and procreation are fundamental to the very existence and survival of the race'.[7] In the intervening years, with the development of the concept of 'privacy', the scope of the fundamental rights doctrine has been even more broadly articulated (as in the abortion decisions). Thus, there would seem no doubt that the kinds of limitations on reproduction which would be needed to achieve the desired genetic effects would deprive individuals of fundamental rights.

The question then becomes whether the state's interest in the result being sought is 'compelling' enough to justify such incursion on personal freedom. If the state were able to show that failure to follow its order would impose a crushing burden on society (or, more grandly, on the survival of mankind), a compelling interest would probably be shown. This throws us back to the issue which began this subsection: namely, whether or not any accurate predictions can be made about future genetic desirability and whether (given mutation) the steps the state proposes to take are likely to achieve the ends sought. Clearly, statements about any rational connections between means and ends are very difficult to make in this field. Usually, there would be no question that the reduction of disease is an end which may be sought through various public health measures.[8] But how far can this be carried? Must the disease that the state proposes to limit through genetic manipulation be lifethreatening, or merely expensive? What burden must it be shown to impose on affected individuals, or on society as a whole? How certain must we be of the genetic mechanism behind it and of its pattern of inheritance? (That is, compare autosomal recessive diseases with multigenic ones or chromosomal translocations.) I would suppose that a programme to eliminate all future offspring with myopia would meet with different reactions than one designed to prevent the birth of children with diabetes or with Tay-Sachs disease; the contrast is further

---

[7] *Skinner* v. *Oklahoma*, 316 U.S. 535, 541 (1942). The Supreme Court held that Oklahoma's involuntary sterilization statute violated equal protection clause since it applied to repeated larceners but not embezzlers, yet lacked any indication of difference in heritability of the two manifestations of delinquency. *But see Buck* v. *Bell*, 274 U.S. 200 (1927) (sterilization of imbecile upheld).

[8] *See, e.g., Jacobson* v. *Massachusetts*, 197 U.S. 11 (1904) (compulsory smallpox vaccination upheld).

drawn if the condition in question is multiple polyposis of the large intestine or a propensity (apparently genetic) to develop nephritis or arteriosclerosis.

Conclusion

I have chosen to discuss the 'legal issues' of genetics in terms of potential conflicts among the various participants in decision-making because it seems to me important to remember that although we are speaking of medical procedures designed to 'help' and 'cure' there are some interests which will have to be sacrificed to achieve ends which may be beneficial to other interests. I doubt that the law, or any other means of mediation, will ever be able to eliminate such conflicts and sacrifices, but it may make us attend to such conflicts and sensitize us to the value decisions implicit in their resolution. It may even, if we are lucky, help to minimize the harm they cause.

References
CAPRON, A. M. (1972) Genetic therapy: a lawyer's response. *In* Hamilton, M. (ed.) *The New Genetics and the Future of Man.* p. 133. (Eerdmans Pub. Co.: Grand Rapids, Michigan.)
—(1973) Legal rights and moral rights. *In* Hilton, B., Callahan, D., Maureen Harris, Condliffe, P. & Berkley, B. (eds.) *Ethical Issues in Human Genetics: Genetic Counseling and the Use of Genetic Knowledge.* Fogarty International Center Publication Proceedings No. 13. p. 231. (Plenum Publishing Corp.: New York.)
DEVLIN, P. (1965) *The Enforcement of Morals.* (Oxford University Press.)
HART, H. L. A. (1961) *The Concept of Law.* (Oxford University Press.)
JONES, O. W. (1972) A new era for cytogenetics. *Current Problems in Paediatrics.* **2,** 3.
RAMSEY, P. (1972) Genetic therapy: a theologian's response. *In* Hamilton, M. (ed.) *The New Genetics and the Future of Man.* p. 157. (Eerdmans Pub. Co.: Grand Rapids, Michigan.)
TEDESCHI, G. (1966) On tort liability for 'wrongful life'. *Israel Law Review.* **1,** 513.
US DEPT OF HEALTH EDUCATION AND WELFARE. (1971) Institutional guide to DHEW policy on the protection of human subjects.

CHAPTER 13

Genetic consequences of abortion

E. Matsunaga

Department of Human Genetics,
National Institute of Genetics, Mishima, Japan

Abortion is a word which is used, often charged with emotion, to mean various phenomena and procedures in different contexts. Since this symposium is devoted to a discussion of genetics and the quality of life, I will confine my usage of the word to mean therapeutic abortion in the context of family planning and population control.

Selective abortion based on prenatal diagnosis is clearly a very refined method of family planning to improve the genetic quality of children, and no doubt this will find wider and wider application in developed countries where a modern family pattern of few but healthy children already prevails and a high level of medical care services is available. On the other hand, we must not forget that in many developing countries the quality of life of future generations depends heavily upon the extent to which the present generation can successfully limit family size so as to halt the rapid growth of population within a reasonably short period of time. For example, most countries in Asia, where more than half of the world population is now living, are characterized by high birth rates and are faced with serious problems arising out of poverty in general; the gap between the living standard of these countries and that of the developed countries is widening, cruelly frustrating their hopes for development. Under the current rates of population increase, it is expected that the total requirements for future health, education, housing and many other welfare needs are bound to increase beyond the capacity of many developing countries in Asia. However, the problems of population growth are not limited to the developing countries only. In some highly advanced countries, the movement toward stabilization of population is becoming increasingly of concern from the viewpoint of the quality of life and the quality of the human environment. In addition, as pointed out by a Report of the Committee on Church and Society of the World Council of Churches 'population growth in the developed countries multiplies their already disproportionate consumption of the world's resources, again frustrating the hopes of the developing countries for a better share'.

Induced abortion is by no means a preferred method of family planning, nor is it the optimal means of population control. Nevertheless, the expert consensus is that abortion may be the most widely used method of birth control in the world, although in recent years, use of the pill and IUD has greatly expanded (Ross *et al* 1972). Recently, the Central Committee of the International Planned Parenthood Federation has stressed that 'the use of reversible contraception alone seems inadequate in most communities to control human fertility within the goals set by many individuals in the modern world', and 'induced abortion plays a significant role in the control of human fertility and is an important factor in the decline in birth rates, especially in urbanized industrialized communities' (IPPF 1972). Thus, induced abortion will continue to have a place in family planning as well as in population control, since contraception alone will never ensure 100 per cent effectiveness. It is therefore of great importance to inquire what kind of genetic changes may occur by widespread use of this procedure. I will discuss this point first and then deal with the case of selective abortion based on prenatal diagnosis.

Genetic consequences of widespread use of abortion
Formally, induced abortion could exert a genetic influence, either directly through: (1) the induction of genic and chromosomal mutations; (2) selection upon the genotypes of the foetuses aborted; or indirectly through (3) changing parental age and family size. Of these, item (2) will be treated in a later section.

Possible mutagenic effect of abortion
No studies have been conducted to see if induced abortion itself has a mutagenic effect upon the oocytes. Pregnancy interruption may or may not disturb the balance of hormones that influence ovarial function. If there were such a disturbance, it might affect the ageing process or the tendency of the stocked ova to chromosomal aberrations. However, judging from the fact that variations, both in the number of preceding pregnancies and in the length of the interval free from pregnancy, have virtually no effect upon the chance of birth of a child with Down's syndrome (Penrose 1934; Beolchini *et al.* 1962; Newcombe and Tavendale 1964; Matsunaga 1967*a*), women having had induced abortions several times are not likely to become predisposed, if the well-known effect of maternal age is eliminated, to bear children with the Down's syndrome in later pregnancies.

Impact of legal abortion upon fertility
In order to discuss the genetic effects of abortion through changing parental age and family size, it is pertinent to examine the extent of the impact upon fertility of the provisions of legal abortion. It is well known that where abortion has been legalized and widely used, birth rates have declined sharply. 'It is in primarily abortion situations (Japan, Central and Eastern Europe) that the most dramatic changes in births over short periods of time have been observed' (Ross *et al.* 1972). In Japan, for example, the birth rate dropped from thirty-four to seventeen per 1,000 during the ten years since the legislation in 1948 of the Eugenics Protection Law which permitted abortion for social as well as for medical reasons. It should be noted, however, that the 1948 level reflects the post-war baby boom, the level of the early 1940s being about thirty-one. During that period the mortality rate also dropped from fifteen to eight. On the other hand, the abortion rate per 1,000 women of reproductive age sharply increased to a maximum of fifty in 1955, but thereafter it has been slowly but steadily declining to twenty-five in 1970, while the birth rate has remained almost constant. According to official statistics, in about 95 per cent of cases the operation was performed within the first trimester of pregnancy. These findings indicate that abortion as the major means of family limitation has been increasingly replaced by contraception (Matsunaga, 1967*b*; Muramatsu 1967).

While Japan's experience must be quite unique, the changing patterns of fertility, induced abortion and contraception (*Fig. 13.1*) fit the model suggested by Requena (1969) well: this model illustrates three stages through which a society may pass, from no birth prevention, through primary reliance on abortion, to major reliance on contraception with some residual abortions to meet contraceptive failure. It should be remembered, however, that in Japan the trend toward lowered fertility has been emerging since around 1920 (Matsunaga 1966). It may well be said that the abortion law in 1948 has merely accelerated this trend.

Genetic effects of changing parental age patterns
In the course of a demographic transition such as that outlined above, a trend is likely to emerge for child-bearing to be concentrated between the ages of twenty and thirty years. The effect of this trend is well known to be beneficial to the health of mothers and their children as measured by indices such as maternal mortality and morbidity, foetal wastage and neonatal mortality. In addition, it is obviously of eugenic relevance, because it reduces the occurrence of new mutations that are correlated with parental age. There are strong positive associations of

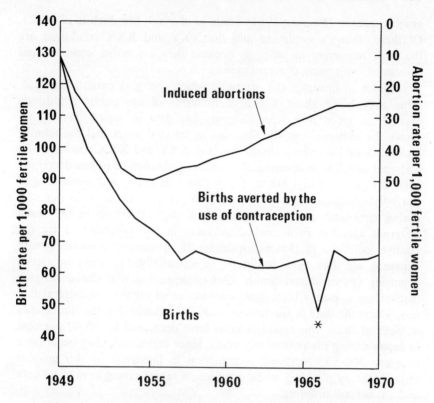

* Ruled by an old superstition: girls born in 1966 were believed to marry unhappily.

Secular changes in the birth and abortion rates per 1,000 fertile women in Japan, showing the increasing use of contraception. Abortions are referred to those notified. Data are based on Annual Vital Statistics from the Ministry of Health and Welfare.

Fig. 13.1

maternal age with the occurrence of certain chromosomal aberrations: Down's syndrome, Klinefelter's syndrome (XXY), triple X female, 13-trisomy and 18-trisomy syndromes (Penrose 1964; Court Brown *et al.* 1969; Lenz 1970). Further, paternal age is known to have a profound influence on the mutation rates for certain dominant conditions: chondrodystrophy, acrocephalosyndactyly, myositis ossificans and arachnodactyly (Penrose 1961; Tünte *et al* 1967; Murdoch *et al* 1972). Of these, Down's syndrome and the XXY and XXX conditions are the most important in practice, because they are rather common and associated with mental retardation.

In order to illustrate the extent to which changing parental age patterns may bring about a benefit in terms of the public health, an example is given here from demographic data in Japan. *Table 13.1* shows the maternal age distributions in selected years and the relative incidences of Down's syndrome and the XXY and XXX conditions by maternal age. The proportion of mothers aged nineteen or less decreased from 2.7 per cent in 1948 to 1.2 per cent in 1968, and mothers aged thirty-five or more decreased from 14.3 per cent to only 4.3 per cent during the same period, resulting in a slight decrease in the mean maternal age, but in a marked decrease in the variance. As for the relative incidence of Down's syndrome, the pattern of association with maternal age has been found to be essentially the same in eleven countries (Penrose and Smith 1966), suggesting that the underlying mechanism is purely biological, irrespective of ethnic and cultural factors. Using the data in the table, it may be deduced that the frequencies at birth of these abnormalities must have decreased by 30-40 per cent in Japan during the past twenty years. Since collectively they occur once in every 300-500 newborn, a reduction in incidence by this amount through family planning would represent a major saving in medical care and in human suffering.

Another genetic effect of changing parental age pattern is related to the reduction in certain congenital malformations that occur in association with maternal age. Since maternal age is correlated with birth order, there will also be some reduction in the incidence of Rh-erythroblastosis and of those malformations for which the risk increases with increasing birth order. Congenital malformations known to occur in association with either maternal age or birth order are, among others, cerebral palsy, strabismus, congenital malformations of the circulatory system and of the nervous system and sense organs. There are no special risks, except for injuries at birth, to children of very young mothers provided they are the first-born (Newcombe and Tavendale 1964; Newcombe 1964). I have estimated that, based on the relative incidences of these malformations and the demographic change in Japan between 1947 and 1960, the reduction may have been about one half for Rh-erythroblastosis, and one tenth for the congenital defects mentioned above (Matsunaga 1966). Since these malformations are caused by many genes in combination with environmental factors, the reduction in their incidence means that the intensity of selection against the genes

Table 13.1

Changing maternal age patterns in Japan since 1948 showing
percentages of births of certain trisomy syndromes

Year	Maternal age							Mean*	Variance	Relative incidence of	
	—19	—24	—29	—34	—39	—44	—49			Down's syndrome	XXXY and XXX
1948	2.7	25.7	30.5	21.8	14.3	4.6	0.4	28.7	37.8	100	100
1958	1.1	27.6	44.4	19.6	6.0	1.2	0.1	27.3	21.9	70	75
1968	1.2	25.2	49.2	19.6	4.3	0.5	0.0	27.1	17.8	61	70

* Calculated using central values of the 5-year intervals.

will be relaxed. However, so long as the same parental age patterns continue, the incidence of the diseases would remain at the reduced level.

Genetic effects of patterns of changing family size

Changes in family size brought about by practising family limitation may have genetic effects in a variety of ways. Trends toward smaller family size will necessarily reduce the frequency of consanguineous marriages by chance, because fewer children mean fewer relatives. Since consanguineous marriages lead to the increased risk of illness, premature death, and congenital abnormality in the children, a reduction in such marriages would reduce mortality and morbidity in the community. For example, if the average mortality of children from first-cousin marriages is double that of children from unrelated parents, and if the frequency of the first-cousin marriages decreases from 5 per cent (which it is in some urban areas in Japan) to 1 per cent, the reduction in death-rate for the population may be about 4 per cent. On the other hand, a decrease in consanguineous marriages should result in an increase in the number of rare excessive genes in the gene pool. However, the rise in the gene frequencies would be very slow and its possible long range effect is not predictable.

Of much more importance is the problem that arises when the same trend occurs with different speeds in genetically different groups. The practice of contraception usually spreads more rapidly in some social strata or groups than in others, and more rapidly among better educated than among poorly educated groups in the society. This would, in all probability, result in fertility differences, and if these were correlated with genetically determined traits, such as intelligence, the gene pool would be altered in a dysgenic direction. In this respect, legislation on abortion laws and availability of facilities seem to play an important role. If termination of pregnancy, not to mention contraceptive services, is readily and equally available to all women who need it, in every class of society, then a fertility differential could probably be minimized, whereas if it is more accessible to the well-to-do than to the under-privileged, the difference would be expanded. In Japan, there is some indication that the fertility differential between social strata has been rapidly decreasing (Matsunaga 1966).

Stabilization of population and relaxation of natural selection

Finally, I wish to discuss the problem of relaxation of natural selection when a population is approaching a stationary state with low birth rate and low mortality rate, the average number of live births per married woman being a little bit higher than two.[1] Natural selection takes place through differential fertility and differential mortality among different genotypes. If each couple had the same number of children that could survive and procreate, natural selection due to genetic differences between families would be removed, only the component due to within-sibship differences remaining, so that deleterious genes produced constantly by fresh mutations would gradually accumulate in the gene pool. While the theoretical aspect of this point will be treated later, in relation with selective abortion, it is highly improbable that differential fertility would completely disappear in human populations.

Table 13.2 gives some demographic data from Japan, showing the change in the fertility pattern of married women during the last thirty years. It should be noted that the figures for women born in the years 1896-1900 refer to completed fertility, whereas those for women born in 1923-27 and in 1928-32 refer to the status at the ages of forty-five to forty-nine and forty to forty-four years, respectively. However, since reproduction by women aged forty years and over has become almost negligible in this country (*see Table 13.1*), the figures for the three cohorts may be comparable with each other. A strong tendency toward a family pattern of two children has resulted in a decline in the mean number of live-born from 5.0 to 2.3; even more marked is the decrease in the variance from 9.0 to 1.1 during the same period. Based on these data, the index of selection intensity for fertility component may be calculated according to Crow's formula: this is the ratio of the variance of the number of parity to the square of the mean number of parity (Crow 1958). This value has decreased from 0.35 to 0.22. This does not, however, necessarily imply that selection for genes related to high fertility or selection against genes causing sterility has been relaxed. One has to recall that the index itself provides only the upper limit, and not the net intensity of genetic selection. It is clear that most cases of sterility in earlier times were due to non-genetic causes such as tuberculosis. Likewise, the sharp decline in recent years in the proportion of women with high fertility is obviously due to cultural rather than biological factors. The population may therefore in all probability not lose its variability as to fecundity and could resume high fertility if social needs required this.

On the other hand, selection through differential mortality has been certainly relaxed by modern improvements in medical care services,

---

[1] According to the latest statistics (1973) from the Institute of Population Problems, the gross and the net productive rates for Japanese woman have been held at around 2.1 and 1.0 respectively since 1956.

Table 13.2

Changing fertility patterns of married women, husband present, in Japan

No. of children ever born	Per cent distribution of number of children ever born to		
Women born in	1896–1900	1923–27	1928–32
0	9.4	6.6	5.6
1	7.6	11.2	13.4
2	6.9	30.5	43.4
3	8.3	29.6	27.4
4	9.9	14.5	7.6
5	11.4	5.4	1.9
6+	46.5	2.2	0.7
Total	100.0	100.0	100.0
Mean (x)	5.0	2.6	2.3
Variance (V)	9.0	1.7	1.1
V/x^2	0.35	0.26	0.22

particularly by the remarkable decline in infant mortality in many countries. In Japan, for example, the infant mortality per 1,000 new-borns was as high as sixty-two in 1948, but declined to thirteen in 1970, a level close to the lowest in the world. The index of selection intensity due to infant mortality may be calculated using another formula by Crow: this is the ratio of the mortality to the survival rate. This value has dropped from 0.066 to 0.013 during the past twenty-two years. Unless environmental conditions become worse and worse because of notorious pollution over this country, the low mortality is likely to persist in the future. But the question of the nature and the extent of its possible long range impact upon society is difficult to answer, since the evaluation depends also upon an environment whose change may not be predictable. At any rate, selective abortion based on prenatal diagnosis will have an important place in a stationary population.

Genetic consequences of selective abortion

Intrauterine diagnosis can now be made, using amniocentesis, of the sex of the embryo, of chromosomal aberrations (for example, Down's syndrome) and many biochemical disorders determined by autosomal recessive genes (for example, Tay-Sachs disease and Hurler's syndrome) or X-linked recessive genes (for example, Hunter's syndrome and Lesch-Nyhan syndrome). In addition, it is possible, by means of ultrasound techniques or amnioscopy, to recognize certain congenital malformations (for example anencephaly) (WHO 1972). Although the number of hereditary diseases that can be diagnosed prenatally is increasing, those likely to come into consideration from the point of view of the application of selective abortion generally lead to pre-adult death of the patients. Further, the fraction of the population that receives any genetic counselling is minute. For these reasons, a direct impact of selective abortion on the gene pool would be small. However, selective abortion may have indirectly some dysgenic consequences if reproductive compensation took place, that is, if the parents, often encouraged, have another child to replace the one aborted, because such a child, although phenotypically normal, may carry a harmful gene in heterozygous form or a translocation in a balanced state.

There are two instances in which selective abortion might follow prenatal diagnosis. The first is the case in which at least one parent carries some kind of genetic anomaly detectable at the genic or chromosomal or phenotypic level. The second is the case in which neither parent has such an anomaly; for example, the embryo may be 21-trisomic in a mother aged over forty years or the foetus may be anencephalic in a mother who has previously borne such a child. In the following discussion, I will ignore the second instance, because it has in practice little or no impact on the gene pool.

Autosomal dominant diseases[2]

The potential effect of selective abortion on the frequency of harmful genes is the greatest and, at the same time, eugenic when it is directed against autosomal dominant diseases with normal or nearly normal fertility, such as Huntington's chorea. If prenatal diagnosis could be made of a dominant disease with regular inheritance in every couple in which one partner is affected, and if all the abnormal foetuses detected could be aborted, the incidence of the disease at birth could be reduced, in only one generation, to a level twice the mutation rate. Though, at

[2] Disease due to a deleterious dominant gene on the autosomal (non-sex) chromosomes.

the present time, no dominant diseases can be detected by amnio-centesis, it may well be possible to recognize by direct observation such dominantly inherited malformations as cleft hand or cleft foot. Further, based on information concerning linkage between myotonic dystrophy and the secretor locus for the ABO blood group substances, it may be possible, by testing amniotic fluid for the secretor status, to assign this disease to the foetus with a high probability (McKusick 1971).

Rare autosomal recessive disorders

In the case of rare autosomal recessive disorders, the effect of any selection is very small and the gene frequency changes only slowly. As a simple model, I will consider a rare recessive disease which leads to pre-adult death of the patients and I will assume that every couple produces two children. Let the recessive harmful gene be a with a frequency of p in the gene pool and its normal counterpart be A. Then there is only one type of mating $(Aa \times Aa)$ from which an affected child with a probability of one in four is born. Since the frequency of such matings is approximately $4p^2$, the incidence of affected children at birth (x) is p^2 prior to the introduction of selective abortion. If selective abortion based on prenatal diagnosis could be initiated in each of these couples after one affected child has been born, and if full reproductive compensation were introduced, that is, if the mother continued to reproduce until she has two normal children, the value of x would be reduced to $\frac{7}{8}p^2$ in the next generation. Thus the reduction in the incidence at birth of affected children would be by 12.5 per cent of the original value.

However, because of reproductive compensation by the births of phenotypically normal children, of which two in three on average are heterozygous (Aa), the frequency of the harmful gene would increase in the gene pool. It is reasonable to assume that, if there is no such compensation, there is a balance between a decline in the frequency of the gene due to loss of homozygotes (aa), that is p^2 per generation, and a gain due to fresh mutation. If full reproductive compensation were introduced, this decline would decrease from p^2 to $\frac{2}{3}p^2$, so that the gene frequency would increase by $\frac{1}{3}p^2$ per generation until a new equilibrium is reached. At this point, the gene frequency would be about $1.22p$ (Motulsky et al. 1971). For example, if the disease in question occurs once in every 50,000 newborn (as is the case with most biochemical disorders that can be diagnosed prenatally), it will take approximately 150 generations, or 4,500 years, for the prevalance of carriers to increase from the present level of one in 110 to one in ninety. Practically, the dysgenic effect of reproductive compensation is no problem in respect to rare recessive diseases.

Rare X-linked recessive disorders

The situation becomes rather complicated with rare X-linked recessive disorders. For the sake of simplicity, it is again assumed that the condition in affected males is so severe that they cannot survive to a marriageable age, and that every couple produces two children. Let the mutation rate be m per locus per generation, then the incidence of affected males at birth among all male newborn (x) is $3m$, of which two in three is the fraction inherited from heterozygous mothers and one in three is due to fresh mutation. If selective abortion based on prenatal diagnosis could be initiated in every heterozygous mother after one affected male has been born, and if the mother continued to reproduce until she has two normal children, the value of x would be reduced to $2.75m$ in the next generation. Thus the rate of reduction in the incidence at birth of affected males would be 8.3 per cent. However, if heterozygous females could be diagnosed in premarital counselling when it is known that at least one of her relatives is affected with the disease in question, the rate of reduction would of course be larger.

Fraser (1972) has studied the possible impact of various strategies of selective abortion on the dysgenic effect of reproductive compensation upon the prevalance of females heterozygous for X-linked recessive genes, and I would summarize here only the most important conclusion drawn by him. If prenatal diagnosis could be made of affected male foetuses (as is the case with Lesch-Nyhan syndrome), so that normal male foetuses could be saved, then, with full reproductive compensation, the prevalence of heterozygous females (y) would increase until after about ten generations it reached an equilibrium point; at this point y will be 1.5 times the original value. On the other hand, if prenatal diagnosis of affected males is not available (as is the case with haemophilia and progressive muscular dystrophy of the Duchenne type), then, based on foetal sex diagnosis, all male foetuses in heterozygous mothers can be aborted. In this case, the consequence differs greatly according to the strategies used, that is whether the carrier females be diagnosed prospectively (prior to marriage) or retrospectively (after they have borne an affected child). If prospective diagnosis of all heterozygous females could be made to monitor each of their pregnancies, so that compensation took place always by the births of two female children, then y would increase by 50 per cent of the original value per generation: it is doubled after two generations, tripled after four generations, and so on, requiring an increasing number of amniocenteses and abortions. However, if the diagnosis were made only retrospectively, y would increase by 50 per cent of the original value after two generations, and by 100 per cent after six generations, but thereafter the rate of increase would become smaller and smaller, the value at equilibrium being 2.3 times the original one. In reality, the diagnosis will be made in some cases retrospectively and in others prospectively, so that the presumed increase in prevalance of carriers will lie somewhere between the two estimates outlined above. Thus, for example, with haemophilia A or muscular dystrophy of the Duchenne type, the prevalence of heterozygous females may increase from the present level of about one in 5,000 to one in 2,500 after two to six generations or sixty to 180 years. An increase by this amount need not cause any serious concern, since there is little doubt that in such a time span, techniques will have been developed for diagnosis of the affected male foetuses.

Translocation carrier

Among a variety of chromosomal aberrations, a balanced heterozygote carrying the t(21qDq) translocation is probably the most important indication for prenatal diagnosis. The incidence at birth of carriers of this type of translocation has been estimated as three in 21,996 $=$ 1.4×10^{-4} (UN Report 1972), and the risk of having a child with Down's syndrome is 10 per cent for female carriers while it is reduced to about 2 per cent for male carriers (Hamerton 1968). If prenatal diagnosis followed by selective abortion of unbalanced heterozygotes could be performed in every carrier parent after one affected child is born, the reduction in the incidence at birth of inherited cases of Down's syndrome would be only a few per cent. However, if carriers could be diagnosed by premarital counselling with reference to his or her relatives being affected with translocation Down's syndrome, the reduction would be much greater. On the other hand, if reproductive compensation took place, the prevalence of carriers would increase.

This point may be outlined as follows:

Assume that premarital diagnosis of all carriers could be made in order to monitor each of the pregnancies, and the mother continued to reproduce until she has two phenotypically normal children. Then the prevalence of carriers in the nth generation, Y_n, would be such that

$$Y_n = (\tfrac{1}{2} + k) Y_{n-1} + 2m,$$

where k is the relative proportion of balanced heterozygotes among phenotypically normal progeny of male carriers, and m is the mutation rate giving rise to a balanced heterozygote of the t(21qDq) translocation. While the value of m has been estimated as $0.6 - 0.7 \times 10^{-5}$ (Polani et al. 1965; Kikuchi et al. 1969), it is still an issue whether or not k is significantly greater than 0.5 (Hamerton 1968; Dutrillaux and Lejeune 1969; Jacobs *et al.* 1970). With $k = \frac{1}{2}$, the prevalence of carriers would increase from the present level of one in 7,000 to one in 5,000 in four generations, and to one in 4,000 in eight generations. However, if k is 0.6, as is suggested by the family data given by Hamerton (1971), the prevalence would increase to one in 3,700 in four generations, and to one in 2,200 in eight generations. It is to be noted that, if carriers were diagnosed only retrospectively, then the rate of increase in their prevalence would become slightly slower.

Needless to say, if, based on prenatal diagnosis, not only foetuses that are unbalanced heterozygotes, but also those that are balanced heterozygotes, could be aborted, the eugenic effect would be as great as in the case of dominant conditions. This raises of course an ethical issue. The above calculation implies that, even if we go without sacrificing foetuses that are balanced heterozygotes, the extent of the possible consequent dysgenic effect need not be of serious concern, at least within several generations.

Summary

Induced abortion, when used legally and widely as a supplementary means for family planning and population control, may have profound genetic consequences through changing parental age and family size, since abortion has been proved to be a powerful depressant of human fertility, especially in urbanized industrialized communities. Data in Japan have shown that the changing parental age pattern must have resulted in some reduction in the incidences at birth of a variety of congentital anomalies that are correlated with parental age and birth order; in particular, the reductions in Down's syndrome, Klinefelter's syndrome and the XXX condition seem to have been considerable.

Changes in family size may have genetic effects in a variety of ways. A trend toward smaller family size by necessity reduces the chance of consanguineous marriages, and hence to some extent reduces mortality and morbidity, resulting in a slow rise in the frequency of rare harmful genes carried by heterozygous persons. Of more importance is that the same trend, if it occurred with different speeds in genetically different groups, would alter the composition of the gene pool. However, if termination of pregnancy, in addition to contraceptive services, is readily and equally available to all women who need it, in every class of society, differential fertility could be minimized. Stabilization of population at low levels of fertility and mortality will necessarily reduce the variation in fertility within population, but not necessarily the variability in fecundity, whereas lowered mortality would relax natural selection through differential mortality, but its possible long range impact upon society cannot be predicted.

Selective abortion based on prenatal diagnosis will have an increasingly important place in family planning where every couple wants to have few, but healthy, children. Its potential eugenic impact on the gene pool is the greatest in autosomal dominant diseases with normal or nearly normal fertility, but techniques have not yet been developed to detect with precision any dominant conditions *in utero*. In hereditary diseases other than dominant ones, selective abortion may have some dysgenic effect if the parents have another child to replace the one aborted, because such a child, although phenotypically normal, may genotypically be abnormal. However, in the vast majority of hereditary diseases that can now be diagnosed prenatally, such a dysgenic effect will in practice be no problem, since they are all rare autosomal recessive conditions for which any selection can change the gene frequencies only very slowly. On the other hand, in the case of rare X-linked recessive diseases and the t(21qDq) translocation, there may be, as a dysgenic consequence, a relatively rapid increase in the prevalence of carriers in the population, thus requiring an increasing number of amniocenteses and abortions. However, the extent of the increase need not cause any serious concern, at least in the forthcoming 100 years.

References

BEOLCHINI, P. E., BARIATTI, A. B. & MORGANTI, G. (1962) Indagini genetico-statistiche sulle fratrie di 432 soggetti mongoloidi. *Act Genetical Medical et Gemellologiae*. **11**, 430.

COURT BROWN, W. M., LAW, P. & SMITH, P. G. (1969) Sex chromosome aneuploidy and parental age. *Annals of Human Genetics*. **33**, 1.

CROW, J. F. (1958) Some possibilities for measuring selection intensities in man. *Human Biology*. **30**, 1.

DUTRILLAUX, B. & LEJEUNE, J. (1969) Etude de la descendance des porteurs d'une translocation t(21qDq) *Annales de Genetique*. **12**, 77.

FRASER, G. R. (1972) Selective abortion, gametic selection, and the X chromosome. *American Journal of Human Genetics*. **24**, 359.

HAMERTON, J. L. (1968) Robertsonian translocations in man: evidence for prezygotic selection. *Cytogenetics*. **7**, 260.

—(1971) *Human Cytogenetics*. Vol. 1: General Cytogenetics. (Academic Press: New York & London.)

INTERNATIONAL PLANNED PARENTHOOD FEDERATION (1972) *Induced Abortion: Report of IPPF Panel of Experts on Abortion* (approved by the IPPF Central Medical Committee). (International Planned Parenthood Federation: London.)

JACOBS, P. A., AITKEN, J., FRACKIEWICZ, A., LAW, P., NEWTON, M. S. & SMITH, P. G. (1970) The inheritance of translocations in man: data from families ascertained through a balanced heterozygote. *Annals of Human Genetics*. **34**, 119.

KIKUCHI, Y., OISHI, H., TONOMURA, A., YAMADA, L., TANAKA, Y., KURITA, T. & MATSUNAGA, E. (1969) Translocation Down's syndrome in Japan. Its frequency, mutation rate of translocation and parental age. *Japanese Journal of Human Genetics*. **14**, 93.

LENZ, W. (1970) Birth defects—genetic aspects. Congenital malformations. *Excerpta Medica International Congress*. Series No. **204**, 402.

MATSUNAGA, E. (1966) Possible genetic consequences of family planning. *Journal of the American Medical Association*. **198**, 533.

—(1967a) Parental age, live-birth order and pregnancy free interval in Down's syndrome in Japan. *In* Wolstenholme, G. E. W. & Porter, R. (eds.) *Ciba Foundation Study Group No. 25: Mongolism*. p. 6.

—(1967b) Evaluation of the family planning programme in Japan. *National Institute of Genetics Mishima Annual Report, Japan*. **17**, 126.

McKUSICK, V. A. (1971) The mapping of human chromosomes. *Scientific American*. **224:4**, 104.

MOTULSKY, A. G., FRASER, G. R. & FELSENSTEIN, J. (1971) Public health and long-term genetic implications of intrauterine diagnosis and selective abortion. *Birth Defects: Original Article Series*. **7**, 22.

MURAMATSU, M. (ed.) (1967) *Japan's Experience in Family Planning—Past and Present*. (Family Planning Federation of Japan, Inc.: Tokyo.)

MURDOCH, J. L., WALKER, B. A. & McKUSICK, V. A. (1972) Parental age effects on the occurrence of new mutations for the Marfan syndrome. *Annals of Human Genetics*. **35**, 331.

NEWCOMBE, H. B. (1964) Screening for effects of maternal age and birth order in a register of handicapped children. *Annals of Human Genetics*. **27**, 367.

NEWCOMBE, H. B. & TAVENDALE, O. G. (1964) Maternal age and birth order correlations: problems of distinguishing mutational from environmental components. *Mutation Research*. **1**, 446.

PENROSE, L. S. (1934) A method of separating the relative aetiological effect of birth order and maternal age, with special reference to mongolian imbecility. *Annals of Eugenics*. **6**, 108.

—(1961) Mutation. *In* Penrose, L.S. (ed.) *Recent Advances in Human Genetics*. p. 1. (J. & A. Churchill: London.)

—(1964) Review of Court Brown, W. M., Law, P. & Smith, P. G. Abnormalities of the sex chromosome completement in man. *Annals of Human Genetics*. **28**, 199.

PENROSE, L. S. & SMITH, G. F. (1966) *Down's Abnormality*. (J. & A. Churchill: London.)

POLANI, P. E., HAMERTON, J. L., GIANNELLI, F. & CARTER, C. O. (1965) Cytogenetics of Downs syndrome (mongolism). iii. Frequency of interchange trisomics and mutation rate of chromosome interchange. *Cytogenetics*. **4**, 193.

REQUENA, M. (1969) Chilean programme of abortion control and fertility planning: present situation and forecast for the next decade. (United Nations, Centro Latin-Americano de Demografia (CELADE): Santiago.)

ROSS, J. A., GERMAIN, A., FORREST, J. & van GINNEKEN, J. (1972) Findings from family planning research. *Reports on Population/Family Planning*. No. 12. (The Population Council, Inc.: New York.)

TUNTE, W., BECKER, P. E. & van KNORRE, G. (1967) Zur genetik der myositis ossificans progressiva. *Humangenetik*. **4,** 320.
UNITED NATIONS. (1972) *Ionizing Radiation: Levels and Effects*. Vol. II.
WORLD HEALTH ORGANIZATION. (1972) Genetic disorders: prevention, treatment and rehabilitation. *WHO Technical Report*. Series No. **497,** 5.
WORLD COUNCIL OF CHURCHES. (1971) *Church and Society—Three Reports*. Study Encounter. 12(3). (Geneva.)

CHAPTER 14

Sickle cell disease — life or death?

A. Eyimofe Boyo

College of Medicine, University of Lagos, Nigeria

This consultation is concerned with the science of genetics and the quality of life which of course can be seen in different perspectives by different individuals and in different cultures. In some cultures, life may be held as being entirely sacrosanct and therefore must be preserved at whatever cost to the individual or society whilst in others it may be considered morally justifiable and indeed humane to eliminate it in those members of society (be they relatives or close friends) whose sufferings are, as a result of disease or injury, considered to be entirely unbearable to themselves and to those around them.

It seems to me that with such a broad spectrum of differing attitudes, some definite position based on ethical, religious or cultural grounds must first be taken before attempting serious deliberation on the impact of genetics on society. I realize of course that a decision of this sort is neither easy nor as clear-cut as it may appear initially. Thus, whilst on the one hand it is considered criminal to harm animals deliberately (particularly those that man has tamed and utilized for his own welfare) in many human societies, it is nevertheless acceptable that a maimed horse or dog for example must compassionately be put to sleep to relieve it of its sufferings. When we deal with maimed human beings on the other hand, we find that we can no longer apply the same ethical compassion simply because we feel intuitively that the right to eliminate a fellow human being on whatever grounds and however justifiable in our opinion or that of others, is one that we cannot arrogate to ourselves.

In most human cultures and religions therefore, there is a serious awareness of the value of and respect for human life as well as a general acceptance of the worthiness of preserving it. When we do deviate from this position then as rational members of the human society we feel the need to provide moral, legal and social justification for the special circumstances that dictated our change of attitude. This is precisely why we are gathered here and indeed why I feel personally that we, and most human beings, regard life as having a qualitative value which cannot be measured by us. In discussing the impact of genetics on society, therefore, we need to remember constantly that none of our preferred solutions should have the attributes of *absoluteness, rigidity* or *permanency*. This is all the more imperative since we know from the history of man that today's solutions may well and sometimes invariably create tomorrow's problems. Man has been evolving for a millenium of years. It would therefore be mere arrogance on our part, particularly with our comparatively very limited knowledge of human genetics, to insist that we have the right to decide in our very short life time the fate of future generations yet unborn irrespective of their own future environment, or to presume that we can control the pattern of the biological evolution of man. All we really can profitably do, is to ensure that nothing we advocate or do in our time shall to the best of our knowledge have long-term adverse effects (social as well as genetic) on the future of man.

It is precisely in this area where political decisions to eliminate life on a massive scale (for example by the explosion of atomic or hydrogen bombs) that man has displayed an utter disregard of the mutagenic effects of his weapons of destruction, and indeed of the effects of his own actions on the genetic endowment which he will pass on to his descendants. To the best of my knowledge the possibility of an increase in the incidence of leukaemias or neoplasia, which medical scientists must have predicted and which indeed did come to pass, was neither considered on ethical grounds, nor even debated, before the decision to let the atomic bomb loose on the cities of Hiroshima and Nagasaki! Political expediency and the right to victory over one's enemies, even though they also be human like ourselves, were the deciding factors.

I have therefore come to be wary of those who continually find the scientist and genetics as the mad ogres of modern society without ever accepting or even realizing that in the final analysis it is the politician and not the scientist who does decide what to do with the products of scientific endeavour. This brief review of the quality of life provides the personal background with which I shall discuss the question of life or death for those who through no fault of theirs have apparently failed to 'choose their parents wisely' and have become endowed with recessive diseases some of which are today regarded as burdens to humanity and to human society.

Ethical considerations

In order for an offspring to be at risk of developing a recessive disease both parents must be carriers of the recessive gene that produces the abnormality although they themselves, being considered as normal, need not necessarily display any overt or clinical manifestations of the disease.

If therefore we are to reduce the incidence of recessive diseases, it is obvious that marriage between, or procreation by, heterozygotes will have to be discouraged or as some would have it even prevented. Yet the marriage between two heterozygotes has the potential of producing *three* apparently *healthy normal* children and only one abnormal child. Working as I do in the environment of a culture which still is considered as being close to nature, I have come to realize two fundamental facts which are perhaps at discord with the Western cultural and educational heritage in which I grew up in my formative years. Nigerian mothers who attend regularly the sickle cell clinics with which I have been associated, range from those with one affected child and three or more normal children to those whose children are all affected. The simplicity of the African way of life makes it possible for the mothers of the first group to accept the simple fact that since not all children can ever be born normal, parents must accept their personal responsibilities and obligations to the abnormal child even when this means regular visits to the clinic. Similarly amongst those of the second group however, I have discovered a strong personal conviction to bear the burden of rearing abnormal sickle cell children, in the full understanding and hope (supported of course by genetic and statistical facts) that their genetic luck will break and normal children will also surely not be denied them much longer. It is unfortunately amongst the sophisticated and Western educated African that I find an unwillingness to accept this latter position. The point I am emphasising is simply that heterozygous marriages not only have three possible chances of having unaffected as against one for an affected child but also that there may well be some moral value and virtue in the acceptance of the infirmities of life. This to me is living—not simply the desire to turn life into a 'bed of roses' in which for the fear of producing one abnormal child we insist on giving up the right to three normal children whose quality of life may well enrich not only ourselves but humanity as a whole.

Not long ago, in thinking aloud along these lines at a meeting similar to this consultation, I posed the question whether human society would have been the richer or poorer if it had been deprived of the artistic contributions of a Van Gogh because his parents having by some miracle gained foreknowledge of his future mental disturbances which were indeed perhaps the creative sources and the inspiration of his art, had voluntarily chosen that he be aborted. Since then, my friend Dr James Bowman in the USA has extended the debate in a recent publication in which he wrote: 'Eugenics is the science (*sic*) of the improvement of humans by better breeding. Many eugenists had a clear and simple solution. Relying upon the new interest and advances in the study of heredity, they felt that the continued evolution of man might be assured by preventing the unfit from propagating and encountering the fit to produce early and often. (Hitler of course, almost succeeded beyond the fondest dreams of many eugenists by loosely interpreting the "fit" and the "unfit" in his "final solution.") Epileptic Dostoevsky and Julius Caesar, drug users Poe and Rimbaud, psychotic Newton and Van Gogh, blind Milton, deaf and son of an alcoholic Beethoven, crippled Kaiser Wilhelm II and Byron, pauper Mozart, tubercular Schubert, Chopin and Robert Louis Stevenson, syphilitic and leprous Gauguin, deformed Toulouse-Lautrec and many others would have been classed among the undesirables according to the 1925 Eugenics Society.'

James Bowman has of course perhaps overstated the case but these men were what they were because of their genetic endowment, their environment and the interaction of both. The point of concern is that in depriving birth right or life to one human being on the basis of a double endowment with a single defective recessive gene, and at the same time refusing the right of birth to three other apparently normal human beings, we are neither qualified nor indeed in the position to determine the extent of deprivation that we may have imposed on humanity as a whole.

This is all the more pertinent when we come to realize that every human being carries at least nine recessive genes which are potentially deleterious in the homozygote and that with advances in the scientific and genetic fields more and more of these abnormal genes will of course come to be recognised with the passage of time. The dilemma is immediately obvious. Are we (as we should do, once we accept social genetic abortion) to offer to posterity a legacy that by all marriages between the many abnormal heterozygotes who, in a matter of years, will become recognisable, should be childless? We might as well face the unacceptable reality that in due course marriage between individuals if dictated by a combination of genetic, social, political and cultural factors will in the future world become near impossible!

It is my view and conviction that in dealing with recessive diseases in particular, we need to assure ourselves that the quality of life transcends human suffering. Our responsibilities and goal should be more in the direction of ameliorating or even finding cures for those recessive diseases like sickle cell disease which really only partially maim and do not deny their sufferer a normal intellectual and near normal physical existence. It is clear that the social solutions for each of these diseases must in fact differ. The amaurotic idiocy and early death within the first five years of a child with Tay-Sachs disease contrast very sharply with the less serious effects of the sickle cell gene in the homozygote and therefore must of necessity receive different considerations.

One very striking and rewarding experience we have had with sickle cell disease in Nigeria is worthy of mention. Less than two decades ago, in extensive population surveys, I, like many other investigators, could not find sick cell homozygotes alive who were older than two years. Today, mainly as a result of the improvement in general health care and delivery and in particular of the philosophy of our own 'keep well clinics' at which patients attend (without any payment of fees) every six weeks whether or not they are ill, the regular use of folic acid and anti-malarial drugs, we have seen afflicted infants through school, university and a useful meaningful life. This debunks the earlier assertions (which even I shared) that the sickle cell gene is lethal in the homozygote, who therefore dies before puberty and is apparently under a sentence of imminent death.

At this point may I be forgiven for quoting in some detail the social facts about a female patient of mine who is now in her mid-thirties, is happily married to a non-sickler and the mother of two normal beautiful children. Before she consulted me she had been seen by a physician and wrongly diagnosed as homozygous sickle cell disease. Her family had been told that she only had a few years to live as she was then in her early teens and in secondary school. She consulted me at this point and with facilities better than those of her physician, I was able to make a correct diagnosis of sickle cell-beta-thalassaemia disease. I took over her management and saw her safely through secondary school—during a period in which incidentally she had a spontaneous splenectomy. She came top of her class in the Cambridge school certificate examination. She did better in this examination than did her younger normal sister a few years later and was awarded a scholarship for further training abroad. Here again her medical history caught up with her and she was nearly refused (but for the persistence of myself and a few others) the scholarship she had won on merit on the dubious grounds that she was potentially a bad investment and a poor medical risk.

Needless to say, she completed her training abroad in excellent time and returned to hold two most responsible jobs in the service of her country. Today she is a happy mother who has had the opportunity to live a useful and profitable life. I know many normal persons for whom this claim cannot be made. We human beings invariably of course hope for a life of at least 'three score and ten' but we do know from experience that this is very often denied a number of us. What I consider to be important is not the length of the expectancy of life of any one individual but the fulfilment of that life to the benefit of the individual as well as society, however short it may be. Dinu Lipatti died in his early thirties of leukaemia and so did Catherine Ferrer (of cancer) at the prime of their lives and musical careers. They left the world a legacy the richness of which many people who have lived their full three score and ten years could never match.

Most of our children with sickle cell disease who often lose a good number of days of attendance at school, do in fact continue to do well and often stay with the upper half of their classes. The contribution which innate intelligence and the intensive parental (particularly maternal in our society) care have in deciding this standard of academic performance, I really do not know. For the sake of our present discussion, however, supposing it was not only just conceivable but also definitely foreseen that sickle cell homozygotes were biologically endowed with better intelligence, would we feel so concerned about their birth? I rather think not.

It is clear therefore, that for me, sickle cell disease and any other recessive disease which imposes some degree of physical or physiological limitation without any mental disability cannot justifiably provide on rational grounds serious arguments in support of the prevention of the birth of homozygotes. I can well see that I am now in danger of being accused of arguing for an intellectual *élite* since I have indeed used normal brain function and normal intellectual performance as essential yardsticks for deciding on the question of social abortion of normal foetuses. I plead not guilty. I have insisted on normal brain function simply because the biological evidence supports the view that man's major attribute, putting him above his ancestral ape-brothers, is the possession of an intellectual capacity which has allowed him to develop sophisticated cultures and social ethical attitudes, both of which also have indirectly affected his biological evolution. The concepts of right and wrong, the ability to recognize danger to one's self as well as to others, all derive from the interaction of our intellectual and cultural heritage. Mentally retarded children, however happy and simple they may be, are nevertheless still in grave danger not only of harming themselves but of harming others simply because they are neither socially nor biologically responsible for their actions. I feel therefore that recessive diseases or dominant diseases which lead to idiocy belong to a category all by themselves and require solutions not necessarily applicable to other genetic disorders.

In arguing for the acceptance of the sickle cell homozygote as not too 'abnormal and deviate' and who in my opinion also has a right to life, let me remind you of three basic facts. Firstly, the albino patient

inherits a metabolic disorder which makes it impossible for him to produce adequate pigment. He therefore suffers from the effects of excessive heat and sunlight as a result of a quantitative defect affecting the
synthesis of human pigment. Socially he may find himself an object of
curiosity and ridicule where everyone else is black but to all intents and
purposes he is regarded nevertheless as a normal human being with a
poorly pigmented skin. If he can overcome the social embarrassment
which this often imposes on him in a predominantly black society, all
is well and he lives a fairly normal and procreative life. The same
albino born into a predominantly white (little or no skin pigment)
society passes usually unnoticed and is spared most of the social trials
with which he was faced in the black community. The second consideration relates of course to the issue of absolute and permanent solutions
which I have already raised. If a cure were to be discovered today for
sickle cell disease, no rational person would continue to argue for
selective abortion of sickle cell homozygotes. Of course a number of
diseases of genetic origin which were originally regarded as incurable
can now be cured—or so well medically managed that normal existence
is ensured—diabetes, hypertension, pernicious anaemia and haemophilia,
to name only just a few. To offer selective abortion as a solution for
any of these disorders would now of course be totally unthinkable.

Finally, the third and most significant fact is that every gene does
not exist in isolation but interacts with other genes which may well
reduce some of its adverse effects. In 1956, as a young research worker
I argued ardently for the existence of modifying genetic factors which
might well alter to the advantage of the patient, the clinical expression
of the disease. Today, we know for certain that the interaction of the
hereditary persistence of haemoglobin F (foetal haemoglobin) and that
of the sickle cell allows a near normal life span free of any serious
debility. Since no two individuals (other than identical twins) are
genetically alike it is obvious that it is not possible to predict, with any
degree of certainty, the beneficial modifications which the internal genetic constitution can have in all sickle cell homozygotes. If we cannot
always determine whether the interaction of the sickle cell gene with
the rest of the genes is advantageous or disadvantageous, on what
grounds then can we presume to have the right to prevent the birth of
any one homozygote?

In view of what I have already said, I find it of course extremely
difficult to accept the concept of voluntary sterilization of either sickle
cell heterozygotes or of heterozygotic marriages between sicklers and
the possessors of genes which determine other abnormalities of haemoglobin structure or synthesis (for example, haemoglobin variants other

than sickle cell). The genetic danger is that such marriages run a one in four risk of having children who will have essentially persistently low amounts of haemoglobin in their blood with or without severe illness. They would nevertheless be capable of physiological adaptations of function which can ensure a near normal life if properly cared for.

Biological considerations in the management of sickle cell disease

The recent concern for the victims of sickle cell disease particularly in the United States of America has created a good deal of social and emotional stress particularly amongst black Americans, simply because action directed against the disease was based initially and almost entirely on political considerations and was not really influenced by true biological knowledge of the sickle cell gene. Thus the official equation of the sickle cell trait with sickle cell disease was both revealing and socially disastrous. It is of course imperative that we know all that is presently known about the biology of any genetic disease before taking upon ourselves the responsibility of proferring solutions. What then are some of the most important known facts about the sickle cell disease and other haemoglobinopathies?

Sickle cell anaemia is the result of the inheritance of a double dose of the gene from two parents who are themselves individuals with the sickle cell trait. Sickle cell disease, on the other hand, includes not only sickle cell homozygotes (that is sickle cell anaemia) but also a number of other heterozygotic conditions in which there is an interaction of the genes for the sickle cell and some other genetic abnormality affecting either the molecular structure (that is other haemoglobin variants) or the rate of synthesis of haemoglobin as in the thalassaemia syndromes. The clinical expression of these diseases varies from almost little or no disablement (as in the SF syndrome), through moderately limiting disorder (for example the combination of the sickle gene and a much less deleterious abnormal haemoglobin gene) to severe illness as may be seen in some but by no means all sickle cell homozygotes. With such variation in the clinical patterns of the disease, it is obvious that a serious consideration of its management must be based on detailed biological and social knowledge of each individual case. Facilities for achieving this level of competence in the diagnoses of the disease are still relatively poorly developed in those very parts of the world where the sickle cell gene is common. The few centres of diagnostic excellence which are to be found in West Africa for example, cannot for the moment provide the opportunity for wide-scale diagnostic involvement in the entire population at risk. The incidence of the sickle cell trait in parts of Nigeria is as high as 25 per cent.

Another biological point of significance is that carriers of the sickle cell gene are normally free of anaemia or any major disability and are in fact no different as far as normal health is concerned from normal individuals. The abnormalities of hyposthenuria and transient haematuria which occasionally occur in some sickle cell carriers are neither debilitating nor particularly disturbing. The most important consideration is that most sickle cell heterozygotes, if not all, are neither anaemic nor likely to suffer from any of the usual complications (for example, cardiomegaly with or without heart failure, thrombotic episodes and so on) often seen in sickle cell disease. It is therefore particularly disturbing that in the USA sickle cell heterozygotes have in many instances been regarded as abnormal and have had special restrictive insurance policies imposed upon them. In this context it is absolutely important that we decide what we regard as disease and what may well be abnormality in some function of the body which does not necessarily comprise a disease state. The claim has often been made that sickle cell trait individuals are at greater risk of dying earlier in life than normal individuals. In America this view has been based on the claims that the incidence of the trait is significantly lower in the elderly (that is the long surviving individuals) than in young adults. To accept this as proven it would be necessary to satisfy ourselves of the complete absence of bias in the methods of sampling of the two groups. We would also need to establish near identical environments for normal and sickle cell trait individuals.

The association of the sickle cell trait with increased risk to survival under certain abnormal physiological conditions (for example high altitude flying and extreme hypoxia) or with morbidity from certain diseases have been used to classify these individuals as abnormal or diseased. When examined in depth however one finds that these claims have often not been based on clear cut controlled scientific enquiry. I know of a number of heterozygotes who have successfully flown as pilots even in the Second World War without any adverse effects. It is of course to be expected that under conditions of severe oxygen deprivation not usually encountered in normal life, the risk of intravascular sickling and hence the induction of intravascular haemolysis or thrombosis would be very much increased in carriers of the sickle cell trait. So incidentally would the risk of cardiac infarction increase under the same abnormal physiological conditions, in persons who appear healthy but who may well have some degree of cardiac insufficiency, under these severely abnormal conditions. Extreme stress of any kind (even emotional stress) may well determine for all of us humans the borderline between normality and abnormality.

Recent studies in our laboratory have shown that abnormality of haemoglobin structure in the heterozygote does not seem to affect adversely its function or that of the red cell. Thus we have recently found that the metabolic production of heat by red cells which is grossly abnormal (that is very much increased) in sickle cell anaemia is in fact normal in the sickle cell heterozygote and practically almost identical with that of normal red cells. Protein structure of course determines the function of proteins but it would appear that the interaction of 25 per cent sickle with 75 per cent normal adult haemoglobins in the red cells of sickle cell heterozygotes does in fact have a protective effect against the adverse effects of sickling which does ensure normal erythrocytic function.

Further, the biological evidence does in fact support the view that in malarious areas, sickle cell heterozygotes are at an advantage in early life and enjoy biological viability which is superior to that of either the normal homozygote with normal haemoglobin or the abnormal homozygote with only sickle haemoglobin in the red cells. There is also strong suggestive evidence on the basis of our work in Nigeria and those of others that marriages between normal and sickle cell trait individuals often tend to be more fertile than those between either sickle cell carriers or between normal individuals. Similarly the infantile mortality appears to be lower in the union between heterozygous sicklers and normal homozygotes than in the latter two types of marriages.

So when we speak of the sickle cell gene as having deleterious effects, this can only necessarily be so for the sickle cell homozygote. The biological effects of balanced polymorphism and heterozygotic vigour in ensuring the survival of sickle cell heterozygotes are determinants which cannot be ignored in the discussion of the genetic welfare of human society.

Finally we need to remind ourselves constantly that no one gene is either good or bad but that each gene has both advantageous and disadvantageous effects. Which of these two may predominate in any one phenotype is invariably determined by the interaction between environment (internal and external) and the entire genotypic constitution of individuals.

Political and social considerations

The USA is the one country in the world to have embarked on a massive programme to eradicate sickle cell disease. In doing so, it has unwittingly reopened some of the wounds of the social injustices of racial prejudice which seem to have plagued America and the American way of life for so long. It has been claimed by some that the political decision to declare a war of eradication on sickle cell disease was to a great extent dictated by the political considerations of an election year as well as the militancy of black power movements which had come to define sickle cell disease as a black man's disease for which the whites will neither find a cure nor with which they will be concerned. Looking at the American scene from the far away shores of Nigeria, which fortunately has a cultural heritage based on the belief that although human beings may have differences in their biological endowment, their right to equal opportunity and to the good life remains unquestionable, one often tends to show both a lack of sympathy and an utter bewilderment at America's racial tragedies.

The truth of course is that sickle cell disease is not racially determined, but as Linus Pauling showed, is a genetic defect affecting the molecular structure of haemoglobin. Haemoglobin occurs in the red cells of all human beings. The sickle cell deficit occurs in some Africans (and indeed in some parts of Africa only), amongst Greeks and other Mediterranean European populations as well as amongst certain groups of Indians. It is even likely that the mutation may have occurred in many other parts of the world in which the selective pressure of malaria was absent and it has therefore failed to survive.

It is unethical of course to impose mandatory laws which demand mass screening of blacks alone, as has been done in certain states of America, when in fact the historical evidence as well as the biological, suggests that even whites may also be at risk. I saw my first *white* case of sickle cell disease at Johns Hopkins through the kind courtesy of Professor Conley. He was blond, fair and blue-eyed and yet he had inherited his sickle cell gene, if I recollect rightly, from a Greek ancestor on the one hand and his abnormal haemoglobin D from an Indian ancestor on the other—no black African ancestry here!

The only tenable position therefore is that if one must screen for heterozygotes for any recessive gene, then one must screen all human beings irrespective of their racial origins. The world as we know it has been in existence for millions of years and human beings have been in social contact for as long as we care to remember. Genes know no racial barriers when transmitted from parent to offspring of whatever ethnic origin and on the basis of Mendel's laws of inheritance. Their frequencies do vary from one human group to another, but that is no basis for refuting the possibility of their existence in members of the human race as a whole.

It seems to me that with the resources of the USA, mass screening should be directed principally towards the identification of diseased sickle cell homozygotes so that they can be offered free and better medical care as we, with our limited African resources have been able to do in a very small way. With regular supervision, the free offer of anti-malarial drugs, folic acid and antibiotic therapy whenever indicated, we in West Africa have been able to preserve the lives of sickle cell homozygotes and to reduce to the minimum its adverse effects.

The amount of money and resources which a mass screening of all Americans white or black would entail could best be diverted to this more rewarding goal.

Of course it seems almost unnecessary to have to remind ourselves that genetic screening should be voluntary and in no way mandatory. The mandatory laws which have so far been passed in the USA on the ticket of good intentions but misguided biology, must be removed from the statute books if we are not to revive the bogey of eugenic racial discrimination which in this day of man's achievement should have been dead and buried in the past.

In conclusion, let me say briefly that I do believe that genetic counsel-ling has an important part to play in the management of sickle cell disease and allied disorders. However, it is my own personal conviction based on our experience in Nigeria that each individual case must be treated on his or her own merit and appropriate genetic advice offered. I have been in the position of realizing over and over again that the need for a normal child in a family whose children so far are all affected, may be so great that it would be ethically wrong to deny them the opportunity of striving for a normal child and taking that one in four chance yet again. In contrast, however, the family with a number of normal children and their first afflicted child should receive the advice not to push their luck further and indeed should be encouraged to feel thankful for their good fortune so far.

All I have said may be summed up in that old adage that 'the possession of a little knowledge is a dangerous thing'. We need to be humble and accept that, as of now, we know so little of our entire genetic make-up that we have great need of being cautious about tampering with it.

PART IV

Genetic Counselling

CHAPTER 15

Psychological issues in counselling the genetically handicapped

Miles F. Shore

Department of Psychiatry,
Tufts University School of Medicine, Boston, Massachusetts, USA

It is necessary that a consultation on genetics and the quality of life should consider psychological factors in work with the genetically handicapped since genetics touches the most sensitive of personal concerns—self-esteem, mental and physical capacity, and procreation. For purposes of discussion, we must define our subject broadly to include those who suffer from physical or mental impairment which is genetically based, their parents and relatives, and those who are genetically at risk. Health professionals who work with genetic problems must settle certain psychological issues to achieve the necessary compassionate objectivity. And the community at large which surrounds handicapped individuals has its own set of psychological reactions which affect the quality of life of these persons.

I have chosen to focus on 'psychological issues' rather than 'psychiatric problems' since our concern is the *quality* of *life* which implies an emphasis upon the enhancement of potential rather than simply the correction of problems. We are thus in the area of *health* rather than the *treatment of illness*. In psychological terms we are concerned with coping and patterns of adaptation, rather than maladjustment, symptomatology and psychological defences. Just as Mendelian principles underly the inheritance of both normal adaptive phenotypes and maladaptive or abnormal ones, so modern psychological principles apply to normal adaptive behaviour as well as to neurotic symptoms. This is an important step both theoretically and in clinical practice, for as we shall see, it is an understanding of this fact which enables us to do preventive health-oriented work with our patients. Of course psychiatric problems do arise in relation to genetic handicaps but there are a great many reactions which are highly creative solutions to complex human difficulties—triumphs of human psychological potential over the extreme vicissitudes of life. And both fall into proper perspective if viewed in the context of coping and adaptation.

In what follows I have chosen to highlight several situations through which we can elucidate principles which are useful in understanding the psychology of the genetically handicapped.

Normal mourning and the family of the defective child

Counselling the genetically handicapped begins with the family—if possible during the pregnancy, but always as soon after birth as the defect is recognized (Tips *et al.* 1964). It necessarily includes the parents as they react to what is inevitably a stressful event (Caplan 1960). The patient's siblings and other relatives may be involved and in some cases the broader community must be included in ameliorative efforts (Lynch 1969).

Denial of the reality or the significance of the handicap is frequently the sign that alerts the physician or social worker to the need for family counselling:

A father sits happily holding his severely retarded five year old son who is unable to walk, stand or sit unaided. The child cannot speak and he has repetitive myoclonic seizures. The child's mother devotes her full time to exquisitely detailed care of the boy, neglecting her seven year old daughter who is rebellious and in danger of dropping out of school. The father, when asked about the son, says cheerfully 'Fred is such a good little fellow, we'd like to have another one just like him'.

This is the kind of case which catches the eye of health workers who mobilize their resources to work on the denial itself. In fact the denial is the visible outcropping of a basic psychological mechanism which is central to understanding the parents of the handicapped. This basic mechanism is the normal grieving process or, more precisely, the process of change of emotional attachments.

When someone or something we care about is lost, there follows a sequence of psychological and physiological reactions which was first described in detail by Erich Lindemann (1944) who studied the relatives of victims of the Coconut Grove Fire in Boston in 1942. The first step in this acute reaction is denial—'Oh no, there must be some mistake'. This is followed by awareness of the loss with a feeling of emptiness, sighing and crying, exhaustion and poor appetite. There is a preoccupation with the deceased and a moving away from other people. Commonly there is an internal search for fault—'What could I have done to prevent this happening?' This acute reaction soon settles into grief work or mourning in which there is a prolonged review of the relationship with the deceased. One by one as they arise, the points of emotional attachment are confronted and the reality of the loss is confirmed with a release of tears. The first work day after her husband is buried the wife sets the alarm clock for 6.30 A.M. then realizes this is not necessary because her husband will never again get up at that hour to go to work. She cries as she has the thought, and the reality of his death is affirmed in relation to that piece of their life together. So he dies a step at a time in her emotional reality. In the course of this process both positive and negative feelings arise. At points where there were irritations or angry feelings the dislike must come up as well as the love. The negative feelings must be experienced and acknowledged or else the emotional attachment will not be loosened. Thus in ambivalent relationships with strong feelings of both love and hate the process may miscarry. When the anger cannot be faced, the attachment remains which leaves the mourner stuck at the stage of denial or chronically depressed or with a variety of psychological symptoms.

When mourning is over the bereaved has felt the reality of the loss point-by-point. The fact that there is no longer an emotional attachment is affirmed and the potential for making new relationships builds up until, like static electricity in a cloud, it is ready to send out a spark. There is a realistic evaluation of the old relationship. The bad has been forgiven and the good appreciated and emphasized. The bereaved is ready then to resume life through new emotional attachments.

This same basic process underlies the reactions of the parents of children who are born with handicaps. As Solnit has pointed out, most mothers during pregnancy expect to have a perfect baby and at the same time fear that it may be defective. The birth of a handicapped child poses two psychological problems: the mother has lost the perfect child which she expected; and she must now come to terms with, and care for, the defective child which she feared. There are of course very realistic aspects to both of these problems. But there is also, in both, a surcharge of the irrational, for the wish for perfection and the fear of defect in the child are partially rooted in the individual psychology of the mother—especially the configuration of her own self-esteem and her mastery of irrational guilt. To understand a particular mother's reaction it is necessary to have information about her own psychological development, the family constellation, and of course, the nature and cause of the handicap if that is possible. In any case, the reaction to the handicap involves a process of mourning or normal grief. There is an initial stage of denial in which realistic planning or effective action is very difficult (Solnit and Stark 1961; Holdaway 1972; Graliker 1959). Emotional turmoil with a sense of disappointment, helplessness and personal failure, is a part of this early phase, for the mother has been unable to create the perfect child she wished for. Being personally invested in what she has produced she may feel as damaged as the child.

The work of grieving takes place as the mother goes over her expectations for the perfect child she did not have. Recall of what she had hoped for and dreamed must be accompanied by emotion—sadness, disappointment or anger. Guilt, irrationally attached to the event, may have to be reviewed and dispelled.

A mother whose son was born with congenitally short arms and deformed shoulders felt she might have caused it because, while pregnant, she had a fierce argument with her mother-in-law and, in a rage seized her by the shoulders to shake her (Lussier 1960).

These irrational interpretations of what has happened are especially important for they may form the locus of an arrest in the grief work. This work takes place in private thoughts, in conversations with friends and relatives and, of course, in contacts with health professionals. It is a natural process which is supported by custom in most societies and it can proceed without excessive professional manipulation. However interruptions do occur. The process may be deflected by guilt or hostility and show up as over-solicitousness or rejection of the child (Graliker 1959; Solnit and Stark 1961). Some parents wish to get pregnant again immediately, ostensibly to make up for the damaged child but really to avoid the work of grieving. This is especially true if the child has died or if there are no normal siblings. In other cases, depression persists and is unrelieved.

An understanding of the expected course of grieving can make it possible for health professionals to enhance the normal mourning process and recognize incipient arrest. Grieving is a repetitive process which takes up to six months. Parents need repeated opportunities to re-examine the loss by talking about it over and over. 'Shopping' for added medical opinions may be a part of the process. To the extent that such 'shopping' is harmful it may be avoided by offering parents the opportunity to review the whole situation repeatedly with the same physician or the team. In contrast, the physician who expects the issue to be settled emotionally in one or two visits is unaware of the true nature of grieving.

Fundamental to the task is a relationship of trust with a counsellor to provide an atmosphere in which it is comfortable to express the disappointment, guilt, and confusion over the child who might have been and the fearful realities of diagnosis, prognosis and management of the child who is. Medical personnel can assist by listening, by acknowledging, and by clarifying as much of the reality as possible. Neither they nor psychiatric counsellors should promote psychodynamic insights in this early phase. Instead, the emphasis must be on support, clarification of reality, and time—all to further the mastery of the experience.

All of this assumes medical personnel are experienced and comfortable with their own feelings. But frequently the physician or others involved in the care feel helpless to deal with the situation. This anxiety may surface as prognosticating too surely, recommending too strongly or expecting parents to function sooner than they can because of their emotional turmoil. Under these circumstances it is difficult for the professionals to help the family do its grief work. Instead the family may be shut off and left to pursue an unnecessarily prolonged course of grief or one which reinforces family pathology. Advice to place a child too quickly may further distort the process. Premature pregnancy to replace the defective child may load the new baby with problems displaced from its predecessor. Genetic counselling during this period before the grief work is done is less likely to succeed because of the recipients' emotional turmoil. Failure to consider this factor may account for some of the discouraging reports of the effects of genetic counselling (Leonard *et al.* 1972).

Normal grief is applicable as the model for understanding the psychology of parents of handicapped children up to a point. But there is one significant difference—the handicapped child remains as a living reminder of the trauma and through the handicap, the child poses new and continuing stresses related to continually disappointed expectations. As developmental landmarks arrive, the parents must adjust their hopes to a level appropriate to that child. Thus the clear resolution of the grief reaction cannot be an invariable outcome. Olshansky (1962) has described the 'chronic sorrow' which is often unexpressed but is nevertheless present in the parents of mentally defective children. He distinguishes it from depression and emphasizes that it does not preclude joy and satisfaction at the achievements of the limited child. It is chronic sorrow which is related to the reality of the handicap and it cannot be wished or 'therapied' away. He wisely admonishes professionals to accept chronic sorrow as part of a reasonable outcome for the parents of handicapped children. Thus the resolution of the grief work for these parents differs in this important respect from the usual outcome of the process.

Psychological development and the handicapped from birth

But I that am not shaped for sportive tricks
Nor made to court an amorous looking-glass; . . .
I, that am curtailed of this fair proportion,
Cheated of feature by dissembling nature,
Deformed, unfinished, sent before my time
Into this breathing world, scarce half made up, . . .
Why I, in this weak piping time of peace,
Have no delight to pass away the time,
Unless to see my shadow in the sun
And descant on mine own deformity;
And therefore, since I cannot prove a lover,
To entertain these fair well-spoken days,
I am determined to prove a villain.

(Shakespeare, *Richard III,*
Act I, Scene I)

Shakespeare's *Richard III* makes clear the sense of outrage and entitlement which he feels because of the intrinsic nature of his deformity. Although no rigorous studies have been reported there is considerable agreement in the literature about the specially personal nature of genetic conditions (Lynch 1969). Freud (1916) identified a group of patients he termed 'the exceptions' who felt themselves to be free of the usual scruples and constraints because of congenital injury. The entitlement to special treatment was justified by the 'unjust disadvantage' which they felt because of their condition. This special status may be reinforced by society. Traditionally the congenitally injured have been ascribed special powers as shamans or soothsayers. Wilson (1941) used Sophocles' *Philoctetes* to epitomize the artist whose creative gift and incurable wound are inseparable.

Although this intrinsic quality is significant, the most important influence on the psychology of the genetically handicapped comes from the fact that the handicap usually exists from birth and thus exerts an important influence on the developing personality.

If grief work is the psychological leitmotiv for the parents of the handicapped, sense of worth and self-esteem is the theme for the genetically handicapped themselves. In childhood the substrate of self-esteem is the structure and function of the body (Greenacre 1958). All of us must struggle to establish a comfortable self concept because as children we are small in size in a big world. Overcoming these normal feelings of inferiority is one of the tasks of psychological development. It takes place through increasing physical proficiency and dexterity as well as by normal growth. Children feel worthwhile to the extent that they can keep up with their peers in running, playing, and other physical skills. Self-esteem is more difficult to attain if the body is misshapen or does not function properly.

A few cases of genetically handicapped individuals have been studied in sufficient depth to shed light on the relationship between personality development and the defect.

Lussier (1960) reported the intensive treatment of a thirteen-year-old boy with congenitally short arms, deformed shoulders and hands with three fingers. Although he was referred for treatment because of enuresis and school problems, the information which emerged in the course of treatment illustrates the way in which his personality traits functioned to overcome the threat to his self-esteem posed by his deformity.

His mother reacted with horror to his birth and blamed herself for the handicap. She did not like to handle him as an infant and found it difficult to enjoy him as he grew up. He was a bright, extremely energetic child whose conversation was full of extravagant claims concerning his prowess. He felt impelled to indulge in daredevil behaviour which was dangerous. For instance he insisted on learning to ride a bicycle although his parents were sure that he would be injured. He became a swimmer and diver against their better judgement. Most importantly he decided that he wanted to be a professional trumpet player. He had dreams of glory in which he was playing the trumpet in front of a huge, enthusiastic crowd.

The purpose of this behaviour was, consciously and unconsciously, to 'prove to the world that whatever anybody else could do with normal arms he could do as well or better with short arms and without artificial aids'. Within himself he attempted to deny the reality of his handicap and built instead a fantasy world in which the handicap did not exist.

Extravagant fantasies of this kind often work against real accomplishment. As a substitute for actions, they can be the basis of serious disruptions of contact with reality. But this boy used fantasy as a precursor of activity. Having dreamed of playing the trumpet he was able finally with great effort to convince his parents that he could be a musician. As soon as he actually had the instrument he abandoned his daydreams about music and threw himself into learning to play.

In contrast to many disabled individuals who use their feeling of entitlement to inactivity to forge an accommodation with the world, this boy was aggressive and energetic and put his 'dreams' to the test. The happenstance of his high energy level shaped the form of his adaptation which, with the help of intensive therapy, had a good outcome. At each stage of his personality development, the handicap, or more properly, his neverending denial of inferiority and perpetual compensatory strivings were an organizing force. As is so often the case successful activity generated reinforcement from the environment. The boy's mother began to take pride in his accomplishments, and for the first time enjoyed him wholeheartedly.

The strength of his underlying wish to undo the handicap made a final bow during the termination of treatment. In separating from the therapist he brought up his disappointment that their work together had not resulted in the growth of normal arms. It is probable that this patient will continue to struggle throughout his life to live out his wish to be just as good (that is as intact) as all the others. And it seems likely that it will be a relatively successful struggle.

Lussier's patient illustrates the effect of deformity on self-esteem in which other personality functions are able to compensate successfully. There are cases in which the handicap itself is so severe that it affects the development of basic cognitive processes which are necessary for personality functioning. Onwake and Solnit (1961) have reported the case of a congenitally blind girl who began a specialized form of intensive therapy at the age of three-and-a-half. She refused to walk, talk, or touch objects. Like Helen Keller she had wild tantrums when her mother moved out of her range. She behaved like an autistic child with a very limited set of pleasures and a distant, mechanical attitude to her siblings and other family members. A careful evaluation showed that her motor and intellectual capacities were normal and so a treatment programme was started.

Over a course of five years of intensive work, it became clear that the absence of visual imagery had made it difficult for this child to organize her sensory impressions in coherent patterns. The results were several. She had no 'stimulus barrier' in the form of a logical conception of the world and was thus prey to a flood of anxiety when confronted with sensory impressions which she was unable to place in a context with meaning. Further, she had no conception of the meaning of her blindness and its relationship to other people. Her questions revealed the problem:

Why can't I write with my eyes? Why did I always want to touch my mother? Where does the loving go when the scolding comes in the voice? Can you see the echo come back? What color is it when it is blue?

Her mother was depressed and overwhelmed at the birth of a handicapped child and the nurse who raised her in the first years was sure that she was hopelessly retarded. Consequently she had a deficit in the close tactile relationship with a protective adult which can help blind children to compensate for the lack of visual imagery. Treatment, which at first included a great deal of tactile stimulation, provided a substitute for this experience and it was thus possible to observe, delayed, the course of personality development. A crucial experience for this child was her awareness of her handicap. As she began to understand that she was blind, and what blindness meant, her chaotic world began to make sense to her. She began to feel a reassuring logic and coherence in her experience. Her terror diminished and her capacity to learn and to relate to other people increased apace. This child's crucial experience was similar to that described by Helen Keller (1961) in her autobiography when language became available to her:

I left the well-house eager to learn. Everything had a name, and each name gave birth to a new thought. As we returned to the house every object which I touched seemed to quiver with life. That was because I saw everything with the strange, new sight that had come to me.

While the emphasis so far had been on the handicap and the adaptive potential of the child, parents play a part in the process of coping. A comparative study of the parents of schizophrenic, neurotic, asthmatic, and congenitally ill children showed that the parents of psychiatrically disturbed children had the greatest incidence of psychological symptoms themselves (Block 1969). The parents of congenitally ill children were described as mature, warm, and responsible, with a striking capacity to sustain and support their youngsters. Of the three groups, the congenitally ill children were most free of psychological symptoms. This kind of study says little about health, that is the psychological mechanisms through which adaptations take place. But it does emphasize the role of parents in enhancing or interfering with coping.

A case study by Kaplan (1959) reports the psychoanalysis of a twenty-eight-year-old man with a right-sided hemiparesis since birth. Although he represented a triumph of physical rehabilitation he sought treatment because he had been unable to marry or to find work commensurate with his level of intelligence. Although these are common reasons for referral for psychoanalytic treatment, in this case they could be traced to the indirect effects of his handicap in which his parents' attitudes had been an important element.

His mother had always felt sorry for him and babied him until he was into adolescence and beyond. His father experienced the hemiparesis as a personal blow to his own pride and turned his feeling of affront into intense involvement in his son's rehabilitation. He would bully him to get him to work on the exercises and other parts of the rehabilitation regimen, and spent considerable time himself massaging his son's limbs. Conforming and rebelling simultaneously, the boy developed a generalized passivity and self-deprecation which made it difficult for him to separate psychologically from his parents and achieve success on his own. This is a frequent response to disability and illustrates the opposite pole from Lussier's patient who was so aggressive and energetic in his adaption. A preventive approach with this patient would have started with his parents. Counselling the mother would have been aimed at helping her to accept the reality of his condition without the pity and sadness which made her try to do too much for him. One can guess that the father may have had some self-serving expectations for a son, or some personal insecurity which was exacerbated by the birth of a crippled child. This personal involvement might have been explored with the father so that he could decrease his persistent efforts to do too much for his son. The boy's own capacity to do for himself could thus have been freed and supported and his character deformity moderated.

Genetic counselling and the psychology of defectiveness

Any discussion of psychological factors in genetic counselling must take into account the great variety of genetic conditions, their varying influences upon susceptible individuals, and the range of human motivations which underlie the decision to seek genetic counselling. The psychological needs of parents with one hemophiliac child who are trying to decide about another pregnancy are very different from those of a twenty-two-year-old recently engaged man whose father has newly confirmed symptoms of Huntington's Chorea. In all cases, the psychological strength and vulnerabilities of the people involved are central factors in determining the outcome. To list these would be to abstract a treatise on personality functioning for they cover the entire range of possibilities. Despite the real diversity there is at least one common thread which runs through experience with genetic counselling. It is the *psychology of defectiveness* which is in constant interplay with the actual threats posed by genetic conditions.

A leading theme in psychological development is a sense of unworthiness which arises in connection with socialization processes in childhood. As children come in conflict with parental and cultural expectations about behaviour they feel guilt or shame as though something were wrong with them. This is easily generalized because of the immaturity of early childhood thinking processes so that children can feel that they are *totally* bad in situations where *one aspect* of their behaviour is being criticized by their parents.

An eight-year-old girl slyly eats a candy bar which her mother had asked her to save until after lunch. When her mother scolds her for being defiant she becomes sad, weeps and says 'Nobody likes me; I'm a bum; I'm no good'.

The exact form of this 'bad seed' concept varies in different cultures and in different individuals. In Western societies which rely heavily upon guilt for behaviour control, the tendency to experience irrationally exaggerated guilt feelings is common. In certain personality types it appears as a feeling of being unlovable; in others as being evil and sinful; in still others as being flawed, defective and not admirable.

There is a general principle in modern psychology that reality reinforcement of the irrational sequelae of psychological development works against adaptation and serves as an organizer of distress and symptomatology which take on a life of their own.

As part of the process of emotional maturation, a fifteen-year-old boy resented his father and at times wished that his parents would get a divorce or that his father would die. His father developed tuberculosis and two years later he did die. The boy developed a hypochondriacal neurosis, became fearful of athletics and failed to gain admission to college although he had superior aptitude.

It is the nature of genetic conditions that they are easily viewed as defects which are especially intrinsic to the individual. Thus there is a very easy reinforcement of personal feelings of unworthiness. The 'bad seed' idea is found in individuals and also has its reflection in social phenomena. The myths concerning teratology (Glenister 1964) and the scapegoating of families with obvious or disfiguring malformations (Lynch 1969) are examples on the community level of a phenomenon which is easily observed in individuals.

A thirty-three-year-old schoolteacher came from an uneducated family who had been ridiculed in their neighbourhood. By great personal effort she had obtained an education and was now a highly successful professional person who dressed very well, moved in sophisticated intellectual circles, and had succeeded in living down the past which she deprecated. When she developed the symptoms of diabetes she was devastated because she felt so defective. She failed to fill out a form for a travel fellowship because it asked her to record any 'physical defects'. And she refused to tell her fiance that she had diabetes because she feared that he would not marry her.

Genetic counselling which identifies individuals with genetic defects lends reinforcement to this sense of unworthiness depending upon individual susceptibility. It is added to by the fact that psychologically fantasy and irrationality rush in to fill the vacuum created by uncertainty and equivocation. Many genetic conditions are poorly understood. It is not possible to diagram the lesion, the causal agent, or the exact mode of inheritance. Concepts of probability are poorly understood by many people and are never an adequate substitute for exact knowledge. Thus, like a Rorschach inkblot test, genetic information may act as a screen upon which is projected the salient features of individual anxiety. Denial which is such a hindrance to effective counselling is often related to the emotional turmoil of acute grief. But it is also an expression of the unwillingness of individuals to admit that they might be as defective as they fear themselves to be. The strength of the synergy between genetic reality and psychological vulnerability is attested to by the kinds of adverse reactions which arise—depression, desertion, divorce, and family disruption.

There is currently widespread concern over the ethics of genetic screening which gives people information about genetic traits or defects which cannot be remedied and which causes anxiety and a feeling of stigmatization (Gaylin 1972). The distress is based in part on the psychology of defectiveness. A responsible approach to screening must take into account the psychological facts. To provide information of this sort will stir up feelings in some individuals and certain groups. Failure to provide adequate means to deal with psychological side-effects is an unjustified violation of professional responsibility. Effective safe-guards include adequate advance information and careful preparation of community leaders and community groups. It may also be necessary to provide group discussion methods or the opportunity for individual counselling in those cases where it is needed. Unfortunately information about the incidence of difficulties and the effectiveness of possible interventions is not available. This paper has stressed a preventive approach and the point has been made repeatedly that constructive outcomes can be promoted by judicious use of psychological skills. Genetic counselling is no exception, however there is not complete agreement about the extent to which psychological matters should be included in counselling.

One approach is to accept at face value the manifest reason for referral, to give the facts as accurately as possible, and refer clients for psychological help when there are signs of obvious emotional distress (Stevenson et al. 1966; Murphy 1968). Other counsellors feel that information is less important than the client's reasons for asking and that sensitivity to various levels of concern and to personal involvements are the counsellor's clear responsibility (Lynch 1969). These positions both have their reasonable aspects. The argument goes to the heart of the psychotherapist's technique where the issue is always how much to do with what one understands. Deep understanding must always be accompanied by a clear definition of goals, and by restraint based upon respect for natural psychological processes since these are powerful forces whose direction is toward the mastery of psychological stress. At the same time, one must recognize that serious psychological stresses are involved in even the best outcomes. Important as it is not to dismantle indiscriminately even superficial adjustment, it is also necessary to understand that there is psychological struggle beneath the surface. The subtle interplay between these two considerations constitutes the substance of a sophisticated and responsible approach to counselling the genetically handicapped.

References

BLOCK, J. (1969) Parents of schizophrenic, neurotic, asthmatic and congenitally ill children: a comparative study. *Archives of General Psychiatry.* **20,** 659.

CAPLAN, G. (1960) Patterns of parental response to the crisis of premature birth. *Psychiatry.* **23,** 365.

FREUD, S. (1916) *The Standard Edition of the Complete Psychological Works of Sigmund Freud.* (Translated from the German) Vol. 14. p. 309. (Hogarth Press and the Institute of Psychoanalysis: London.)

GAYLIN, W. (1972) Genetic screening: the ethics of knowing. *New England Journal of Medicine.* **286,** 1361.

GLENISTER, T. W. (1964) Fantasies, facts, foetuses: interplay of fantasy and reason in teratology. *Medical History.* **8,** 15.

GRALIKER, B. V., PARMELEE, A. H. & KOCH, R. (1959) Attitude study of parents with mentally retarded children. *Paediatrics.* **24,** 819.

GREENACRE, P. (1958) Early physical determinants in the development of the sense of identity. *Journal of the American Psychoanalytic Association.* **6,** 612.

HOLDAWAY, D. (1972) Educating the handicapped child and his parents. *Clinical Paediatrics.* **11,** 63.

KAPLAN, E. (1959) The role of birth injury in a patient's character development and his neurosis. *Bulletin of the Philadelphia Association for Psychoanalysis.* **9,** 1.

KELLER, H. (1961) *The Story of My Life.* (Dell: New York.)

LEONARD, C. O., CHASE, G. A. & CHILDS, B. (1972) Genetic counselling: a consumer's view. *New England Journal of Medicine.* **287,** 433.

LINDEMANN, E. (1944) Symptomology and management of acute grief. *American Journal of Psychiatry.* **101:** 141.

LUSSIER, A. (1960) The analysis of a boy with a congenital deformity. *Psychoanalytic Study of the Child.* **15,** 430.

LYNCH, H. T. (1969) *Dynamic Genetic Counselling for Clinicians.* (Charles C. Thomas: Springfield. Illinois.)

MURPHY, E. (1968) The rationale of genetic counselling. *Journal of Paediatrics.* **72,** 121.

OLSHANSKY, S. (1962) Chronic sorrow; a response to having a mentally defective child. *Social Casework.* **43,** 190.

ONWAKE, E. & SOLNIT, A. (1961) It isn't fair—therapy of a blind child. *Psychoanalytic Study of the Child.* **16,** 352.

SOLNIT, A. & STARK, M. H. (1961) Mourning and the birth of a defective child. *Psychoanalytic Study of the Child.* **16,** 533.

STEVENSON, A. C. & DAVIDSON, B. C. C. (1966) Families referred for genetic advice. *British Medical Journal.* **2,** 1060.

TIPS, R. L., SMITH, G. S., LYNCH, H. T. & McNUTT, C. W. (1964) The 'whole family' concept in clinical genetics. *American Journal of Diseases of Children.* **107,** 67.

WILSON, E. (1941) Philoctetes: the wound and the bow. *In The Wound and the Bow.* (Houghton: Boston.)

CHAPTER 16

Ethical problems in genetic counselling

Robert F. Murray, Jr.

*Department of Paediatrics and Medicine,
Howard University College of Medicine, Washington, D.C. USA*

Genetic counselling is one of the oldest forms of genetic intervention in the history of modern medical practice. It was probably practised on a minor scale for hundreds of years before the nature of the gene was even understood.

The earliest genetic counselling was probably given in a non-scientific fashion by laymen to a young man or woman about to marry into a family where insanity or some other familial, behavioural character or disease had been noted. The prohibitions of certain religious groups against marrying very close relatives might have served the same purpose, but such regulations were inconsistent and more often than not male oriented. In Judaism, for example, aunt-nephew marriages were not allowed, while uncle-niece marriages were accepted. These practices were undirected, often unscientific and frequently misguided. However, their effect, in a genetic sense, was probably insignificant.

In modern genetic counselling we give information based upon a presumed knowledge of the distinction between conditions which have major genetic determinants and those which (apparently, at least) do not. And further, we are armed with a battery of clinical biochemical and cytological tests by which we can, in a small but significant number of cases, pinpoint the specific defect. We may then give precise genetic recurrence risks where single gene defects are involved or approximate risks where multifactorial traits or chromosomal anomalies are concerned.

Genetic counselling like medicine is part art and part science. And the counsellor like the physician is invested in an actual or a potential sense with a great deal of power. The medical doctor has, at some level, the power of life or death over his immediate patient and he is sworn by the Hippocratic oath to promote well-being and support life. Most modern physicians adhere to this, although sometimes at excessive economic and emotional costs to the patient and his loved ones. The counsellor in one sense has life-and-death powers. But his influence has the potential for extending from the counselee throughout an entire family to future generations even though this potential power may not be directly or completely exercised. The effect of information given to a couple may be multiplied many times over depending on the counsellor, the method of counselling, the condition involved and the social climate.

Unfortunately, there is no 'genetic counsellors' oath'. Nor is there any standard by which the layman or the counsellee is able to judge the quality of information he receives or the compassion and sensitivity with which it is transmitted. There is no licensing procedure, nor is there at the moment agreement on the minimum standards of training, that is its quality or quantity, which would be required for a person of a particular background to qualify as a counsellor at any level.

The status of genetic counselling might be compared to that of the modern automobile mechanic. He repairs your car and your life depends upon its correct mechanical junction. Yet the automotive mechanic is not logically required to demonstrate his competence. Almost anyone with the temerity to represent him or herself as a genetic counsellor, to whom someone will come for counselling can say that they are, in fact, a genetic (or educational, or biomedical, or biogenetic to give a few alternative names) counsellor. An evaluation of their legal responsibilities suggests that they have none and are not liable for malpractice if they are *not MD's*. In other words, the counselee is not now legally protected from being given false misleading information or biased information by the non-MD genetic counsellor. This may seem at first glance only peripherally related to ethical considerations in genetic counselling, but as I proceed with my discussion I hope to show why I feel the current legal status of genetic counselling is important and in particular 'why the background of the genetic counsellor is important in analyzing the values involved in genetic counselling'.

There are at least two different settings in which genetic counselling may occur which are distinguished by the way the counselee is motivated or brought to seek counselling. The first and best known category is that which operates in standard medical practice.

In this situation the counselee is an individual with an illness diagnosed by a physician as being of genetic origin, or the parents of a child with an illness diagnosed as being of genetic origin seek advice about the risk of having offspring with the same condition. The persons involved in this situation are usually highly motivated and very interested in getting all the available information. They are anxious to be fully informed about the risk of recurrence and to learn all they can about the condition.

In contrast to this is the situation that is becoming more and more common, namely the situation in which persons who are healthy are told that they are at risk to develop disease or otherwise healthy parents are told that each is the carrier of a gene mutation which will not affect their personal health, but which will with a certain probability produce disease in their offspring should an egg and sperm, each carrying the same mutant gene, combine to form an individual. The motivation of counselees in this setting may vary widely from those vitally interested to those who are only curious, or who may have been coerced by social or familial pressure to seek counselling and those who are frankly hostile or negative. Many of these persons have been involuntarily identified in large-scale screening programmes such as those mounted for sickle cell disease. Most (at least 60-70 per cent based on our own survey) who volunteered for testing believed that the test result would be negative in their case (Murray 1974). It is especially difficult for people who are struggling to deal with their self-image as with many American blacks to adapt to the new and unwelcome knowledge that they carry a gene mutation and must also come to grips with the prospect of giving birth to a child who is ill when they have *no* children at all.

Obligations of counsellor to counselee
One focus of the counselling situation is on what the counsellor does to, with, or for the counselee. For the sake of this discussion let us assume that the information given the counselee is accurate. (Some evidence from sickle cell screening programmes suggests that this is not necessarily so.) But what of those other aspects of information transfer that are so vital (Lejeune 1970)?

(1) Is the counsellor neutral or biased regarding the information transmitted? What criteria are being used to determine how and in what amount information is transmitted? Should he impinge upon the freedom of the individual or couple to make their own choice as far as is possible by slanting the statistics one way or the other or should he support their feelings about what they wish to do? For example, Down's syndrome has a one in 50 recurrence risk, but a mother of thirty has a twelve times greater chance of having a second affected child than a woman of her age who has not had a child with Down's syndrome.

(2) Is the counsellor justified in offering advice to the individual or parents, even when he is asked for such advice? If giving biased or loaded information infringes upon the freedom of the patient or parents to choose, the offering of advice by the counsellor will no doubt make it virtually impossible for the counselee to choose otherwise unless he

or she happens to be someone who enjoys rebelling against authority.

Since the physician-counsellor in the medical setting is obligated to do no harm and to preserve the well-being of the patient, his role might be to support the decisions of the counselee, but on the other hand he is also supposed to be interested in relieving or preventing suffering and pain, and not insignificant are the presumed needs of society. Here is where there may be ethical conflict in the physician-counsellor's mind. Which is more to be valued? The freedom of choice of the patient and his social and emotional well-being or the obligation of the doctor to prevent suffering? But there may be suffering of at least two kinds. The very real suffering of patients and parents who receive the bad news of the genetic recurrence risk, especially if the recurrence risk is high because of the anxiety it generates and the potential suffering of that potential second affected child that might be conceived if the parents decide to take the genetic risk.

But no matter what their choice, the physician-counsellor is obligated by his oath to promote the physical and emotional well-being of his patients to the best of his ability.

One might then ask who is the patient in this setting? For the relief of suffering of the immediate patient, that is the counselee, suggests that the potential suffering of the potential patient will take second place.

The doctor-patient contract is an explicit one that is difficult, if not impossible, to break. This can be corroborated by physicians who have been involved in malpractice suits. A recent consequence of the concept of the parents as patient is the rapidly growing practice of amniocentesis. This is the diagnosis of inherited and other defects in the developing human embryo by the study of cells and fluid taken from the amniotic sac surrounding the embryo, followed by therapeutic abortion before twenty-two weeks of those foetuses found to be affected with the biochemical or chromosomal evidence of a genetically determined illness. The stated object of foetal destruction is often said to be prevention of suffering of the foetus as well as the parents. But there is some degree of suffering in any form or condition of human life. This then begs the eternal question of how much suffering is acceptable in human life and who should be the measurer of such suffering? Should this be decided by the physician or the parents or some independent commission? Millions of children without genetic or congenital defect are born into poverty and will suffer just as predictably as children with potential disease. Should we then abort all children born to parents of a certain income? Furthermore, genetically diseased and malformed infants can be destroyed more efficiently by practising infanticide, according to Lejeune (1970) since there are so many disorders that do not become apparent until late in gestation not to mention the many congenital malformations that can only be detected visually or by careful physical examination. Of course, the response made to this idea is that one does not wish to take 'human life' and embryonic life is only 'potentially' human. But isn't *potential* life as genuine as *potential* suffering? The web of this logic or its sophistry becomes more tangled if this line of inquiry is followed. The issues in this setting are fairly clear. The physician-counsellor can take no course of action that does not result in some type of ethical conflict. Unless a 'new' kind of physician is to be created the obligations implicit under the doctor-patient relationship and the physician's continued dedication to the preservation of life will determine the ethical values to be given first priority.

What has just been discussed occurs in the traditional medical setting. The parents involved already have a child or children, one or more of whom is sick. Some element of illness already exists and the counsellor is eagerly sought for aid and sometimes advice in decision-making.

With the advent of simple methods of testing for disease and, in particular, for detecting the carrier state, that is, the condition in which the subject carries in single dose a gene which in double dose will produce disease, has led to some genetic counselling being carried out in a quasi-medical or sometimes even in a non-medical setting. In large-scale screening programmes counselling is being done by non-physicians, nurses, social workers, specially trained family workers and in some places by enthusiastic laymen. Since these counsellors are not physicians and there is no legal doctor-patient relationship, since they are not ethically or legally bound by the same oath or laws that designate the obligations and responsibilities of the physician, the ranking of values involved can be significantly more difficult.

I do not mean to imply that paramedical professionals or highly-motivated and intelligent laymen are not sensitive to human needs for in certain instances they may be more sensitive than the professional. But in the case of conflicting values, the rules governing their resolution of ethical conflicts are less well defined.

Add to that the difference in the way that persons may come into the counselling setting and certain contrasts will become apparent.

Let us consider the childless couple where both husband and wife have been identified in a screening programme as carriers of a serious, either debilitating or painful disease. They have been drawn into the testing programme often by fear, curiosity, pride, loyalty, guilt or perhaps by accident, but seldom because they have experience with the disease in question. Since most don't expect to be found positive, they are therefore ill-prepared for that 'bad' genetic news. The knowledge that theirs is an exceptional situation (one in 144 couples will both carry the gene for sickle cell trait where one in 12 black Americans carries the sickle cell gene or one in 400 couples will both carry Tay-Sachs disease where one in 20 Americans of Ashkenaz-Jewish descent carries the gene for this neurological condition) is of little consolation. Indeed, in some instances, the couple may feel singled out by cosmic forces for punishment as suggested by studies of Fletcher (1972).

But the significant difference is that the counselees who enter the counselling setting are brought abruptly from a position of health, well-being and usually ignorance of the disease in question, to find themselves suffering emotional pain and conflict because of an act that is performed in most cases in the interest of preventing suffering that *might* occur if couples such as this one should have children. The probabalistic behaviour of genes is such that certain of these couples would not have *any* affected children if they went on to have children and most would have no more than *one* child affected with the condition.

If sixty-four couples where both parents are carriers for an auto-somal recessive trait each has three children, twenty-seven would have no affected children, twenty-seven would have one affected child and two unaffected children, nine would have two affected children and one normal child, one would have three affected children (Li 1961).

The worst tragedy is with those less common, yet highly visible cases where two or three affected children are born. Such cases stick most prominently in the minds of medical and especially non-medical people and there is a strong tendency, conscious or unconscious, to discourage childbearing when such couples seek counselling.

The lay counsellor, since he or she does not have the physician's obligation to the counselee as patient, may well adopt the potential child as patient or focus on the potentially unfortunate couple or couples who may have had multiple involved children as patients. Not only might the freedom of choice and well-being of these couples be compromised but their self-concepts and their feeling for one another may be jeopardized and seriously compromised (Fletcher 1972). How does one weigh the loss of the happiness and feeling of self-fulfilment that can come from having one or more children with a chronic and incurable disease for which the couple is jointly responsible and at the same time not directly responsible? What guilt and psychic pain do they suffer when they decide to take a chance and have a child and they are unlucky? Should they be penalized by society because they knew of the possibility in advance, especially when the counsellor does not provide support for their decision? Furthermore, the parents are still subject to the risks of any other couple to have children with birth defects other than the one under consideration.

Such couples have less cause for concern about being forced to have the child if the disease in question can be diagnosed by amniocentesis in early pregnancy and the foetus aborted. This is the case with Tay-Sachs disease where amniocentesis can be performed in couples at risk and cells cultured from the amniotic fluid can be assayed for an enzyme hexoseaminidase A, and the diseased (or potentially diseased child) therapeutically aborted. There is direct application of the genetic information and if the couple has *no* conflict about therapeutic abortion the couple can fulfil their dream of parenthood while the potential suffering of the child with Tay-Sachs disease is prevented. The conflict remaining is the destruction of potential life. One long-term effect of this procedure will be to increase the frequency of mutant Tay-Sachs genes in the gene pool because mutant genes that would ordinarily be lost in affected homozygous children will no longer be removed and there may even be reproductive compensation (Motulsky *et al.* 1971).

In contrast, the couple with sickle cell trait can only be *certain* of avoiding the birth of a child with sickle cell anaemia by *not* having natural children. And the insensitive counsellor may introduce more anxiety, especially for the male, by suggesting that they might have a child that is likely to be free of disease by practising artificial insemination using a donor known not to be a carrier of sickle cell trait or any other haemoglobinopathy. The female member of the couple may be fulfilled at the expense of the oh-so-delicate male ego. It is very interesting that another logical alternative to artificial insemination of the female carrier by sperm from a donor who is known not to be a carrier, is the insemination (artificial or otherwise) of a female who is a non-carrier by the sperm from the carrier male. A discussion of reasons why this alternative is usually not considered might shed considerable light on the relative importance of not only the genetic contribution of male and female but the importance of the womb in which gestation takes place.

To exercise free choice is to risk guilt and suffering of both parents and child. But is a child who is chronically ill of less value than a child not ill (or not obviously ill)? It would appear to be so in our society! The sick child is a person and unless severely retarded mentally very probably experiences most, if not all, human emotions and relates (often in a healthier way) to other human beings. I can see no sound ethical or moral basis for devaluing a child or person with a chronic illness unless the ethical system is economically based. The argument that each person has a *right* to a 'normal' or 'healthy' life does not stand up under close scrutiny. Arguments that would lend support for the idea of wrongful birth would, in my view, also lend support on logical extension for infanticide.

One strong justification for restricted childbearing by my hypothetical couples is based upon the supposed needs of *society* rather than those of parents, patient or child. In this case the overriding ethical considerations are conditioned by the economic costs of a particular course of action or the contribution of a particular course of action to society. But who is to determine those needs and should they be based on utilitarian or humanistic ideals?

Obligations of the counselee to society

It is in this context that I would like to introduce a concept which has been hinted at by some writers but which has not been very clearly spelled out. This is the concept of a 'new' kind of physician whose patient is society rather than a particular individual.

What shall we call our new physician? He might be called social physician or eco-physician or socio-eco-physician. The training for this specialist would be significantly different from that of physicians as we know it including the epidemiologist. Like the modern public health physician he would work for various govenment agencies, but unlike them he would relate only to populations. He would see patients only to get some feel for disease categories but throughout his training would be shielded from developing any concept of or concern for the traditional doctor-patient relationship. This aspect of medical training would be omitted. By law he would be protected from the obligations of the doctor-patient relationship.

What sort of curriculum would he follow?

(1) He would have a strong background in economics.
(2) He would be knowledgeable about population genetics.
(3) He would study intensively ecology and ecological relationships.
(4) He would have to understand demography.
(5) He would have to become quite expert at statistical analysis.
(6) He would have to understand motivational psychology in order to promote certain patterns of behaviour in individuals or particular groups.

The upshot of this modified curriculum would be a physician whose view of medicine would be primarily group and economically oriented. His concern would be the health of the community as a whole which would be promoted by eliminating or preventing the birth of sick or potentially diseased individuals unless it was clear that medical treatment would be economically more feasible than screening and counselling or therapeutic abortion.

Which approach is best?

Since each of us is aware of the obligation of the traditional physician to 'do no harm' and to preserve life and relieve suffering, we know that our welfare is supposed to be the focus of his efforts and his judgements. Might we feel the same way sitting across from the 'new physician'? Are those who feel that we should have as major concerns the composition of the human gene pool or the costs of diseased persons to society or the burden of diseased individuals on society prepared to become patients of the 'new physician'? Would you feel comfortable knowing that the decision of whether or not to treat you, and if so what method of treatment and for how long, was being determined mathematically according to a predominated formula geared to the projected needs of our society rather than those of the individual or his family?

One serious problem with this kind of approach is we know little of the 'true' economic cost of genetic disease and even less about its psychosocial impact. Most cost accounting does not include all the costs of screening and treatment and does not begin to estimate social and emotional costs which are real but are difficult and probably impossible to measure.

Eliminating genes that determine disease might be beneficial from the disease standpoint, but might not be beneficial from an adaptive point of view since the carrier status of the Tay-Sachs or sickle cell genes might confer benefits that are currently unknown. One can readily visualize a society in which the motivation to prevent inherited disease of any sort might become strong enough to make mandatory screening for all possible metabolic and chromosomal disorders as well as the carrier status. Couples where both carried the same trait and who knowingly married and had affected children might eventually be penalized in some way by, for example, having health insurance benefits withheld. The matching of suitably coded IBM punch-cards might become an essential ritual part of the courtship dating game. Cards would be matched and if no holes coincided the couple might proceed to determine whether they might be compatible in other regards.

If they are properly emotionally prepared and there is some *positive* therapeutic or deterrent alternative available for the couple at risk, then voluntary, prospective genetic testing is probably the approach of choice, but because of our state of limited knowledge and our current efforts to humanize a dehumanizing society, physicians and genetic counsellors ought to continue their emphasis on the welfare and obligation to the immediate individual or family.

The gene pool, the community and society are all theoretical constructs made possible by a collection of individuals. History should have taught us that unethical behaviour directed toward individuals almost always has a corrupting influence on society despite the fact such behaviour might be for some higher principle that supposedly supersedes individual values. Recall if you will the result of the French Revolution and the Hitler régime.

If we can only love those humans we value and since we may be moving toward the devaluation of human life that does not meet certain standards of 'normality' one would have to raise serious questions about modern humanism in Western society.

Almost everyone recognizes an inherent 'right to life' but attempts to answer some of the following questions are fraught with conflict:
(1) When is this right irrevocable?
(2) If not, when can this right be revoked?
(3) Does this right apply to all human life? Past a certain stage of development?
(4) Should anyone other than parents or the individual himself decide about the termination of life?
(5) Is the exercise of this right contingent on certain standards of 'humanness'?

Most of these questions are unresolved. Further, we understand little of our complex genetic heritage and how it operates over time. What genetic counsellor has the wisdom, sensitivity, knowledge to be confident even after answering these questions and many others to prescribe for a given couple a definitive course of action? I know of none.

To do *more* than (1) provide as clearly and as sensitively as possible all that we know of a given situation and (2) to support parents while *they* make a decision of a course of action implies (in my mind) an unjustified exercise of power and control by anyone involved in genetic counselling today, and perhaps at any time in the future.

References

FLETCHER, J. (1972) The brink: the parent-child bond in the genetic revolution. *Theological Studies.* **33,** 457.
LEJEUNE, J. (1970) On the nature of men. *American Journal of Human Genetics.* **22,** 121.
LI, C. C. (1961) *Human Genetics: Principles and Methods.* p. 70. (McGraw-Hill: New York.)
MOTULSKY, A. G., FRASER, G. R. & FELSENSTEIN, J. (1971) Public health and long-term genetic implications of intrauterine diagnosis and selective abortion. *Birth Defects: Original Article Series.* **7,** 22.
MURRAY, R. F. (1974) A public health perspective on screening and counselling in sickle cell trait in genetic issues in public health. *In* Cohen, Bernice (ed.) *Genetic Issues in Public Health.* (Charles C. Thomas: Springfield, Illinois.)

CHAPTER 17

Social and ethical problems in caring for genetically handicapped children

Spyrox A. Doxiadis

Institute of Child Health, Athens, Greece

This paper describes only the problems arising in the family and in the community from the *presence* of a genetically handicapped child. Questions of prevention or of genetic counselling for future children by the same parents are not dealt with here. Neither do I go into the very important question of the psychological problems created in the child and in other members of his family since these are described elsewhere in this consultation.

The meaning of genetic handicap

The children we mean when talking about genetically handicapped, are those with chromosomal abnormalities (about five in 1,000) or with inherited metabolic disorders of large effect (about ten in 1,000) or with major congenital anomalies of a complex etiology comprising a genetic element (variable incidence because of varying environmental factors).

We should however, bear in mind that any child may have a genetic make up which may develop into a handicap. I do not mean by this that all of us are heterozygotes for some five to nine harmful genes, because these may harm the offspring of the person who has them, not the person himself.

My meaning is that in the extreme variability of our genetic makeup there are in some persons elements which may lead to physical or mental ill health only under adverse environmental conditions. A typical example from physical health is the common variety of rickets, which is called 'nutritional rickets', indicating that it is due, as everybody now knows, to lack of vitamin D in the body, either because the child does not get enough sunlight or not enough vitamin D in his diet. We came however only recently to realise that not *all* children in a population will develop rickets in the absence of the above factors; and more of these differences in individual susceptibility to environmental factors are being discovered.

More important than these differences in the development of physical illness are the great individual differences in the field of behaviour. It is only in the last few years that by the use of scientific methods in the study of the behaviour of newborn and young infants we realised the great individual variabilities existing in this field. Modes of behaviour, of reaction to stress, to insult or to the environment in general, if not recognised and respected, may lead to mental ill health in exactly the same way as non-recognition of the need by some children of a certain vitamin leads to physical ill health.

This very wide definition of a genetically determined handicap may not be useful in the day-to-day clinical practice; it is however, I think, a concept, psychologically and socially useful. It makes the major handicaps appear only as extreme variations of a normal range, therefore it does not set totally apart the handicapped children. Furthermore it keeps us all aware of the constant interplay between genetic endowment and environmental influences among all individuals, healthy or sick, and it increases our sensitivity to the different needs of every child and our respect for the individuality of every person.

The variety of major handicaps

In order to start thinking about the social and ethical problems created by the presence in a family of a genetically handicapped child a grouping according to etiology is not useful, especially so for non-medical people. What we need is a description of the various groups of handicapped children on the basis of the problems they present for their general care, their education and the outlook for their future.

The following are the main groups as seen by the family, the community, the school, the state:

(1) The severely retarded child, needing almost always institutional care.

(2) The mildly retarded, therefore educable in special schools or in special classes of ordinary schools.

(3) The children with learning difficulties or disorders (as from sensory handicaps—deafness, blindness) needing early detection and special education.

(4) The children needing early detection and constant and diligent care so as not to become retarded. Typical examples are babies suffering from biochemical disorders such as phenylketonuria or galactosemia, who should receive from the first weeks of life and for many years a special diet so that their brain is not damaged.

(5) The children with motor handicaps, but mentally normal or nearly normal (all the variety of cerebral palsy).

(6) The children needing very specialised surgical and medical care for the correction of their abnormalities and still remaining handicapped (for example major abnormalities of the central nervous system such as hydrocephalus).

(7) The children kept in reasonable health with constant medical care but with no chance, at present, of survival beyond puberty. Here the main example is thalassemia major (Cooley's anaemia), perhaps the most important genetic problem in some countries.

Differences among countries and cultures
It is known that throughout history there were, in different cultures and in different periods, varying attitudes as to the fate of handicapped persons. Even within the same period and culture the attitudes varied according to the age and the nature of the handicap. In ancient Greece, for example, a deformed newborn might be exposed to die, while a blind old man was revered and respected.

In the countries and the cultures of today it is worth bearing in mind that the degree of development and wealth may influence the type of problem. With increasing development, meaning more wealth, more industrialisation and more urbanisation there are two different and opposing influences.

The genetically handicapped are favoured by the greater availability of medical and technical services for earlier detection, for prevention, for special treatment. But more development (as development takes place today in most countries and not as we would have wished it to be) acts also against them. This is particularly evident in those children with a mild mental retardation or with a motor handicap. These children can adjust themselves much better in a rural or semirural small community, rather than in a highly competitive, impersonal large city setting, where even transportation requires good physical ability.

Regarding therefore the social care for the handicapped children, the problems in a less developed country or in a small community are different, that is need for better medical services, while in a urban setting the need is for life in a smaller community with less competition and more acceptance of the handicapped, more personal contracts and no need of transportation.

Social and ethical problems
These cover a very wide range, from decisions on life and death, to questions on the quality of life, on allocation of resources, on protection of mental health. Some of these are described here:

(1) The problem of keeping alive a hopelessly retarded child. This is the continuously debated question of euthanasia, no matter if the

cause of gross retardation is genetic or acquired (as mentioned above in many central nervous system abnormalities the etiology is multi-factorial). There is a tendency among clinicians nowadays to agree that although no positive measures to terminate life can be considered, no 'extraordinary' measures to prolong life should be taken. The debate now centres around the distinction between 'ordinary' and 'extraordinary' measures. The giving of fluids and food is undoubtedly ordinary, even the parental nutrition during an acute illness is the same. But what about the need for parental nutrition for months or indefinitely? Is it an ordinary or extraordinary measure? Since it requires a lot of medical and nursing care and when there is no visible end to this need it should be considered extraordinary. Furthermore big surgical interventions are extraordinary. But if they can correct, but only partly, the anomaly as in hydrocephalus and spina bifida—what then? Should one operate, when in some children survival will mean a permanent physical disability in vital functions of the body? There is a lively debate going on now among pediatricians, and two tendencies are becoming recently clear. The first is to get a better understanding, by a longer and more thorough follow-up, of the outcome of various surgical procedures on babies with central nervous system or other severe anomalies. Thus one can define better the indications for active treatment early in life. The second tendency is to assess results, not any more on a narrow physical basis, but on a broader basis considering as well psychological and social aspects of survival, that is the quality of life for the child and his family.

The question of negative euthanasia is too vast to be covered here. There is a need, however, for public discussion in each country, since some of the factors influencing policy may vary from one place to the other as mentioned in previous parts of this paper. There is a need furthermore for a consensus of opinion: on general policy, on definition of terms, on accepting both scientific data and ethical and social aspects as basis for discussion. There is a need, in other words, of education of the public so that it can participate in a democratic way in establishing the general guidelines for the conduct and the decisions of the professionals. Once this has happened the decision for each individual should be left in the hands of a few experienced and competent professional persons, who have got to know the family and the child well, and who should in each case decide whether, or how, the parents can participate in the burden and the responsibility of the final decision.

(2) The problem of not increasing the initial handicap. This is an extremely important family and community responsibility and it is particularly relevant for children with mental retardation of mild or moderate severity and for children with a sensory handicap. The most

important single measure to avoid increasing the retardation is to keep the children in the family and not in an institution. Well conducted observations have shown that institutionalized children with Down's syndrome have, in comparison to those living with their families, significantly lower intellectual capabilities and they score significantly lower on social maturity scales.

Although, as in all clinical and welfare work, each case should be decided separately and after consideration of all factors (parents, siblings, education, finances) we should realise that for most mildly or moderately retarded children, the best place to grow is their home. This, however, will not be achieved or, if realised, will put on the family an intolerable burden unless society provides supporting services. It has been estimated that the cost of even the best services (family counsellor, domestic help, financial aid, baby sitters trained for handicapped children, special day schools) will not be higher, and is usually lower, than residential care (if this is an acceptable standard).

In general lines the same policy is desirable for children with sensory handicaps or other learning disorders.

(3) Related to the above is the problem of continuity and comprehensiveness of medical care. This appears to be a medical problem, but it is social in the sense that society will have to provide funds and facilities for the establishment of special units and teams for the genetically handicapped children. What usually happens today is that the long-term management and the short-term crises are faced by different doctors, without co-ordination or co-operation with the other members of the health or education team.

(4) The problem of *finances*. The cost for the *care* of the genetically handicapped varies widely according to the type of handicap. The cost is not excessive, for example, for children with thalassemia major (Cooley's anaemia) requiring one or two pints of blood every six to eight weeks, nor for the special diet of a phenylketonuric child for a few years. But the question of the cost becomes very important and gives rise to discussions about priorities, when we consider, for example, the cost of keeping a severely retarded or a severely spastic child in an institution for life. Then in all countries, and more so in the poorer ones, the question arises if the limited amount of money available should better be spent for these handicapped children, or for the establishment of a new special unit for heart surgery, or for a school for nurses, or for rural dispensaries. The question of priorities in the allocation of resources has been debated in the last few years in many countries and in many international conferences. My feeling is that we, in the health professions, have been too ready to accept as final the percentage from

the national budget given for health services and we have been only arguing about the better use of this percentage. This is too timid an attitude. I think that, in collaboration with our colleagues concerned with education and welfare, we should be pressing our governments for a larger percentage of the national budget for these three services. We should individually and collectively say that this increase should be at the expense of the percentage allocated to 'defence' which in some countries may mean 'aggression' and in others 'suppression'. Whatever it means it is money spent in preparation to kill. Part of this money should be diverted to improve the quality of life.

(5) The problem of informing the parents that their child has a potential, genetically determined, defect. Here we need clarity on what we mean, because there is a variety of cases with a different degree of risk. There is for example the case of finding in a normal child the XYY chromosomal constitution which has been found more often among criminals. On the other hand it is estimated that there must be thousands of socially normal individuals with this constitution. There is on the other hand the case of the infant or young child in whom we detect by clinical observation or by special tests some characteristics in his behaviour which we assume to be genetically determined and which, if not properly handled, may lead later to behaviour disorders and maladjustment. In this case it is necessary to forewarn and advise the parents because the child can be greatly helped by understanding and proper management. But do we extend this obligation to let the parents know in the first case, that is of the XYY child? Do we help them or the child, or do we create in them constant anxiety and unhappiness which also will inevitably affect the child?

This problem is likely to become more acute and more important as our knowledge on the genetics of behaviour increases as it is bound to do. Today it is considered likely there is a genetic basis for our behaviour and I can only hope that, in the next few years, what is now mostly a hypothesis based on few facts and many surmises or extrapolations, will acquire a respectable scientific basis.

(6) The problem of procreation of the genetically handicapped. We have to know in each particular instance the genetic risk for the children to be born, the risk for them, even if healthy, of growing up under special conditions (if a parent is physically or mentally ill), and the risk of increasing in the genetic pool the number of defective genes. It has been estimated that with treatment of phenylketonuria and ability of the treated to grow up and have children it will take forty generations for the number of homozygotes to be doubled. This last risk is not large enough to create any problem, but surely it is not the same

with more common conditions such as hereditary anaemias in some areas of the world. There are in the Mediterranean area regions where the number of heterozygotes for thalassemia is 7-10 per cent of the general population. The prevention of marriage of two heterozygotes is based on detection and education, not compulsion. What however, would the effect be, if a method of treatment is found by which homozygotes, most of whom now die before or at adolescence, survive till the age of marriage? In this and similar instances what should society do? Has it a right of intervention? How and by whom will it be decided? These are still unanswered questions.

(7) The biggest problem of all is how to make all people feel that the genetically handicapped children are not different children; they may be anybody's children and their care is the responsibility of all of us.

The answer is education of all people as to our responsibilities and this consultation may help towards this goal.

CHAPTER 18

Sociogenetic problems and public opinion

Wilhelm Tünte

Institute of Human Genetics, University of Munster, West Germany

In recent years there has been much debate as to whether the human gene pool will deteriorate in future as a result of increased mutations and relaxed selection. In order to maintain the quality of the genetic endowment, a widening use of some measures hitherto uncommon or even as yet not feasible in human reproduction like artificial insemination, selective abortion, predetermination of sex, and extrauterine breeding has been proposed or predicted. However, the essential question of whether people will actually use these methods, instead of common reproductive practice has not been given due attention. Thus, Crow (1971) wrote: 'The big unknown is man, of course, for the future direction of selection depends on human decisions'.

In an attempt to fill this gap, I carried out a socio-genetic inquiry in collaboration with Dr Benno Biermann, a sociologist, affiliated with the Fachhochschule Münster. At the end of 1971, 2,000 individuals, at least fifteen-years-old, living in Nordrhein-Westfalen, were questioned about their knowledge of some topics in human genetics and their attitudes toward problems in human reproduction raised by recent developments in genetic research. These individuals constituted a quota sample of the population in Nordrhein-Westfalen, selected for sex, age and profession. The inquiry was done by some 100 students of medicine and psychology.

The goal of our inquiry was the elucidation of the following questions:
(1) What do people know of genetic factors as causes of diseases?
(2) What is their knowledge of genetic counselling?
(3) What is their attitude toward the consequences of genetic risks?
(4) Are they willing to accept responsibility for the genetic quality of future progeny?

In the following, some selected results pertinent to this consultation on genetics and the quality of life are presented. In looking at the data, it should be remembered that the findings are based on a quota sample, and that no generalizations should be made. It should also be noted that the figures do not provide information on what people would actually do, but only indicate what people say they would do. Obviously, there will be some correlation between such statements and actual behaviour.

Knowledge of genetic disease

About 80 per cent of all respondents claimed to know a genetic disease. Females seemed to be slightly more familiar with hereditary affections than males. If one takes these figures at their face value, a rather encouraging picture emerges in respect to people's knowledge of genetic disorders. It changes, however, rapidly, when it becomes clear that almost one-third of all interviewed persons denoted such diseases as genetic which are commonly classified as non-genetic (for instance tuberculosis, cancer, varicose veins or speech defect). An additional one-fifth quoted collective diagnosis (mental disease, mental deficiency, blindness, deafness, or lung disease and others) which could not be considered as correct answers.

Of those who claimed to know a genetic disease, only 40 per cent of the males and 45 per cent of the females were actually able to term a hereditary disease. About 20 per cent named a monogenic disease. The best known example was haemophilia, followed by colour blindness, and more rarely, by phenylketonuria and galactosemia. Some 14 per cent mentioned a polygenic disease, in most cases diabetes, schizophrenia or hypertension. Roughly 5 per cent named malformations and some 2 per cent, chromosome disorders. If the number of respondents with correct answers is related to the entire sample, then only about one-third are able to mention an example of a genetic disease correctly.

Knowledge of genetic counselling

A further item was concerned with people's knowledge of genetic counselling. Some 90 per cent indicated that they knew of the possibility of obtaining medical advice about genetic recurrence risks. About one-third of these said that they would apply to the family doctor, an additional one-third would turn to a specialist. Only about 7 per cent of the respondents said they would contact an institution specialized in providing genetic counselling. Two conclusions may be drawn from these figures: in seeking genetic advice a marked majority of the sample would apply either to the family doctor or a specialist. This underlines the urgency of the physicians being familiar with the basic principles of genetic counselling. On the other hand, only a small minority know of genetic counselling as a special medical service available in all institutes of human genetics. This explains the well-known fact that human geneticists in general are rather infrequently asked for genetic advice. Some additional data suggest that a considerable proportion of the respondents would seek genetic advice in institutes of human genetics if they were properly informed. Hence, more adequate information for the public is urgently needed.

The question of whether an abortion should be induced in an unequivocal case of a severely malformed or imbecile foetus, was affirmed by some 89 per cent of the males and 85 per cent of the females (*Table 18.1*). These figures make it clear that a majority of the sample accept pregnancy interruption on genetic grounds. For some people the proportions of assenting votes might appear rather high, sufficiently high to ask whether they might be a peculiarity of the quota sample studied. Two points should be mentioned here. First, the question takes for granted that there is no doubt about the diagnosis of severe damage. This condition may have influenced some respondents to assent to abortion. Second, similar results were obtained in a representative poll conducted by 'Infratest', in March and April of 1971, of the population of eighteen-year-olds and over in West Germany. Thirty-three per cent of the men and the women favoured interruption of pregnancy if it was feared that a child would be born with physical or mental defects. This proportion comes very close to our figures.

The percentage of affirmative votes is higher in Protestants than in Catholics, the figures being about 95 per cent and 83 per cent respectively (*Table 18.1*). This difference was to be expected. Nevertheless, considering the strong opposition of Roman Catholic Church to induced abortion, the percentage for the Catholics seems to be fairly high.

Table 18.1

Question: If there is no doubt that a severely malformed or imbecile child will be born, should the pregnancy be interrupted?

Answers:

	Males (no.=934)	Females (no.=1,066)	Protestants (no.=652)	Catholics (no.=1,274)
no	10.8%	14.3%	5.2%	16.9%
yes	89.1%	85.0%	94.6%	82.6%
no answer	0.1%	0.7%	0.2%	0.5%
Total	100%	100%	100%	100%

Concern for future generations

Another question was aimed at testing people's sense of responsibility for bad genes that do not manifest in their own children and grandchildren, but may impair the genetic quality of future generations

(*Table 18.2*). Some 50 per cent of the men and about 44 per cent of the women said they would have no children at all in such a case. The proportion of those preferring only to limit the number of offspring was somewhat larger in females (44 per cent) than in males (about 39 per cent). Only some 11 per cent of all the respondents said that they would plan the number of progeny, ignoring any genetic risks to future generations. The proportions are almost the same for Protestants and Catholics.

The figures suggest that a large majority of the respondents are willing to accept responsibility for the genetic quality of future generations, even on the premises that their own children and grandchildren will not be affected.

Table 18.2

Question: If you were aware of having undesirable genetic factors which will become manifest not in your children or grandchildren, but in more remote descendants, how would you behave?

Answers:

	Males (no.=934)	Females (no.=1,066)	Protestants (no.=652)	Catholics (no.=1,274)
completely resign to children	49.9%	44.4%	45.9%	46.5%
limit the number of offspring	38.5%	44.0%	42.9%	41.6%
plan the number of progeny independently	10.9%	10.9%	10.1%	11.3%
other or no answer	0.6%	0.8%	1.1%	0.5%
Total	99.9%	100.1%	100.0%	99.9%

Attitude to genetic risk

We also tried to find out the attitudes of the respondents toward a high genetic risk for the offspring, owing to a hereditary defect in the male partner of a couple (*Table 18.3*). Only about 4 per cent of the men and the women wanted to have their own child with their marital partner despite the high genetic risk. Slightly over 60 per cent of both the men and the women said that they would have no children of their own, but adopt a child, and about 30 per cent of all respondents would prefer to have no children at all. Fully 5 per cent would recommend an artificial insemination with donor semen in order to have a child. There are only minor differences between Protestants and Catholics.

The results are informative. The two extreme possibilities, namely a rather conservative one (own child at any price) and a fairly progressive one (artificial insemination with donor semen) are favoured only by some 4 per cent and 5 per cent, respectively. The proportion of stubborn (or quite optimistic?) respondents appears to be encouragingly small. Artificial insemination seems to be favourable only for a small minority, too, because at present it is still charged with strong emotional taboos and many unsettled ethical and legal questions.

Table 18.3

Question: If you were married (for women) to a genetically affected man or (for men) as a genetically affected man and the risk of producing a child with malformations or imbecility would be very high, how would you decide?

Answers:

	Males (no.=934)	Females (no.=1,066)	Protestants (no.=652)	Catholics (no.=1,274)
want a child with my marital partner in spite of the risk	3.7%	4.3%	2.6%	4.8%
resign to own offspring but adopt a child	60.3%	62.0%	59.5%	62.6%
completely resign to children	30.6%	28.4%	32.1%	27.8%
recommend an artificial insemination with donor semen	5.4%	5.3%	5.8%	4.9%
Total	100.0%	100.0%	100.0%	100.1%

Slightly less than two-thirds of all respondents said that they would assent to adoption. This indicates that adoption will probably increase if future genetic counselling is requested by a growing number of couples. Almost one-third would prefer to remain childless.

We studied the question of how the sense of responsibility for the genetic quality of future generations might be associated with the attitude toward abortion on genetic grounds and toward high genetic risks for their own children. *Table 18.4* shows that the proportion of those who argued for abortion on genetic grounds is highest (some 88 per cent) among those who, in the case of transmitting bad genes to future generations, would accept responsibility by completely resigning to children or by limiting the number of offspring.

Table 18.4

Attitude to the risk of transmitting bad genes to future generations[1]	Number of respondents	In the case of a severe physical or mental defect, the foetus should be aborted[2]			
		yes	no	irresolute, no answer	total
completely resign to children	939	87.5%	12.2%	0.2%	99.9%
limit the number of offspring	829	88.5%	11.2%	0.2%	99.9%
plan the number of progeny independently	218	78.9%	19.3%	1.8%	100.0%
other or no answer	14	71.4%	28.6%	—	100.0%

[1] and [2] For precise formulation of the underlying question see Tables 18.2 and 18.1 respectively.

Table 18.5

Attitude to the risk of transmitting bad genes to future generations[1]	Number of respondents	In the case of a high genetic risk for own children[2]				
		completely resign to children	adopt a child	want an own child	recommend artificial insemination	total
completely resign to children	939	32.1%	62.5%	0.6%	4.8%	100%
limit the number of offspring	829	26.1%	63.3%	4.6%	6.0%	100%
plan the number of progeny independently	218	29.8%	48.6%	16.5%	5.0%	99.9%
other or no answer	14	50.0%	42.9%	7.1%	—	100%

[1] and [2] For precise formulation of the underlying question see Tables 18.2 and 18.3 respectively.

A similar but even stronger association is shown in *Table 18.5*. Only 0.6 per cent of those, who would completely resign to children in view of genetic risks for future generations, said that they wanted their own child despite a high genetic risk. The corresponding percentage rises to about 5 per cent in those who would merely limit the number of off-spring. It even increases to almost 17 per cent in those who would plan the number of their progeny, ignoring possible damage to the gene pool of future generations.

The data presented in *Tables 18.4* and *18.5* suggest that most of those respondents who are willing to accept high responsibility for the genetic endowment of future generations, would also take preventive measures if a high genetic risk were given for their own children. The observation that the findings are consistent with each other indicates that the respondents have deliberately given their answers.

Conclusion

The genetic future of man is frequently considered as being threatened by an imminent deterioration of the gene pool, due to increased muta-tions and relaxed selection. This pessimistic view is often based on rather vague conclusions drawn from present developments in modern medicine and technology. It is my impression that the results of such a simple extrapolation from present observations to future events appear less threatening if man's balancing reactions to adverse developments is given due attention. Admittedly, it is very difficult to predict how people will react in future on those events that may alter the quality of the human gene pool.

The sociogenetic inquiry, a few results of which have been described briefly here, presents only a small and rather crude contribution to the study of what people eventually might do when they would have to make decisions pertaining to the genetic quality of their own children or more remote descendants. Our results seem to indicate that a majority of the respondents would decide in a reasonable manner, appropriate to the presumed genetic risks. On the other hand, the findings do show that more information on the characteristics of genetic disorders and on the benefits of genetic counselling is urgently needed for the public. According to my own experiences, people are often more familiar with some future kinds of genetic engineering than with present needs of genetic counselling. This discrepancy ought to be reduced by providing proper information which should be given at school, in public lectures and by the mass media.

In our study healthy individuals have been interviewed for their knowledge of hereditary defects and of genetic counselling and for their attitudes toward some specified genetic risks. This hypothetical background must be considered when the findings are to be interpreted. Certainly, it is of particular importance to find out what people, who are themselves affected, know of the genetic nature and risks of their diseases, and what their attitudes are toward reproduction. In pursuing this goal, we shall interview some 1,500 adult patients with polygenic congenital malformations in order to study the biological and social effects of these anomalies on their lives.

Reference

CROW, J. F. (1971) The effects of a changing environment on man's genetic future. *Bioscience* **21,** 107.

PART V

Findings and Recommendations

CHAPTER 19

Findings on genetics and the quality of life

*As explained in the introduction to this volume the members
of the consultation drew up their findings and recommendations at its conclusion. Their findings follow together with
recommendations which are printed in bold type.*

1. New opportunities and new questions

New possibilities in the application of human genetics present individuals and society with new decisions that have to be made. The possibilities remind us that every achievement of new human powers calls
for decisions about how those powers will be used. When such powers
extend to purposeful acts upon the human genetic constitution, decisions
acquire an intimate and important meaning.

The issues we see emerging are of various kinds. One refers to the
methods currently in use or about to be developed for the correction of
genetic defects. Another concerns the alleviation of suffering of children
inheriting defects and of parents transmitting them. Still another involves
the issues of the modification of the reservoirs of genes, the gene pools
as they are called, in different populations, by eugenic programmes,
whether voluntary or legislated, and by such factors as reduction in
family size.

In considering human responses to genetic situations, we can identify
four factors which must be taken into account. The first of these is the
human values of individuals. The second is the obligation of society to
individuals. The third is the obligation of individuals to society. The
fourth is the question of deciding how to implement measures that are
needed to help individuals make decisions in respect to genetic problems. These factors, taken as a group, raise issues between education
and persuasion, on the one hand, and social pressure and coercion, on
the other—issues to which we shall return repeatedly in this report.

Wherever and whenever possible our knowledge should be used to
provide all children with the capacity for life without severe mental or

physical defects, and a measure of nurture and education that will enable them to achieve a full development of their capacities.

a. *A case study*
Whatever principles we may state, genetic problems are deeply personal and often involve profound conflicts of values and feelings. The following case is presented to illustrate a situation in which the lack of easy solutions to genetic problems may serve as a stimulus to reflection upon the ethical and psychological conflicts which arise in decision-making. No claim is made that the case is 'typical'; in fact, cases are often highly particular and individual.

A thirty-two-year-old woman and her husband discover that she is pregnant for the third time. Several years earlier she had a child who died at the age of three with the diagnosis of Cooley's anaemia, a genetically based blood disease which is fatal before puberty. A second child has just been diagnosed as having the same condition. The woman is three months pregnant. Both she and her husband come from religious families which strongly disapprove of abortion. Furthermore, both of them are highly motivated to have children. Each is from a large family in which family life was defined as important and as including several children. Their brothers and sisters are fertile, and much of the life of the extended family is organized around the presence of children. Their cultural background emphasizes the importance of the 'blood line', as they call it; and having natural children is part of the meaning of masculinity and femininity.

In discussion with a counsellor the options appear this way:

To continue with the pregnancy involves a 25 per cent risk that the child will have the condition. In that event the prospect, even with the best of maternal and medical care, is death before puberty. Both parents' reaction to the death of the first child was prolonged. The mother was depressed for nearly a year and really recovered only when she became pregnant again.

Abortion conflicts with their religious principles, and they anticipate considerable guilt should they choose this option. In fact, they indicate that they really want the counsellor to *advise* them to take this course; they could not bring themselves to take the responsibility for choosing to 'kill our child'. They are afraid that they could never get over the feeling that the child they had eliminated might have been normal. And they sense that this decision would be a decision never to have any more children of their own.

Adoption involves rearing a child who does not carry on their inheritance. No one they know has ever adopted a child and felt right about it. The feeling that adopted children are tainted products of illicit sexual activity is widespread in their cultural group. The mother is not sure that she could love someone else's child.

Because the husband is a carrier of the recessive gene that causes the disease in question, artificial insemination by a donor other than the husband (AID) is mentioned by the mother as a way of avoiding the defect in her children, in a separate interview which she has arranged without her husband's knowledge. He is a jealous man who has never felt particularly sure of himself. His wife is afraid to raise the question with him because she fears his reaction. She herself wants to make a biological contribution to her child, and yet she fears that she would be committing adultery if she had AID. She is fearful that she might be attracted to some other man or might become emotionally involved with thoughts of the biological father.

Such a case study illustrates the interplay of many factors in decisions concerning genetics. There is the need for the most adequate information available. There is the importance of the feelings of the parents, even when those feelings are not shared by counsellors and experts. There are genuinely ethical issues, involving possible conflicts of values. There are human relations between husband and wife, and between the couple and their relatives. There are expectations of society and of the social groups surrounding the family. There are religious traditions and loyalties which the family is re-examining. The presence and interaction of so many forces is a reason why an answer to the family's questions cannot be reached glibly or dogmatically. In these many respects the questions in this case example are characteristic of questions that arise widely as people consider possibilities inherent in new genetic discoveries.

b. *The suffering caused by genetic disorders: avoidance, acceptance and sharing*

One purpose of reducing genetic defects is to reduce human suffering. Although suffering is an inescapable aspect of human life, it can often be avoided or diminished. Genetic disorders may cause suffering through the physical and mental limitations they impose on the patient, even to the curtailing of his life, as well as through the consequent physical, psychological and financial burdens placed on others. The family, the medical profession and society should strive to minimize such suffering whenever possible without violating other moral values.

The avoidance of suffering is not, however, the only value to be sought. Not only is suffering sometimes unpreventable or unremediable. but it may have redemptive value for those who are touched by it. Religious traditions recognize that people, through suffering, can grow as well as diminish, and can discover dimensions of life that would otherwise remain closed. The effort to avoid confrontation with suffering too often leads to human insensitivity and to the devaluation and isolation of those who must suffer.

Christian faith, in particular, acknowledges several aspects of human suffering after the example of Jesus of Nazareth. It seeks to prevent suffering and to heal the sick. It accepts solidarity with those who suffer. And in the inavoidable sufferings of life it seeks the grace that comes through suffering.

c. *The relation between scientific advances and ethics*
Churchmen cannot expect precedents from the past to provide answers to questions never asked in the past. On the other hand, new scientific advances do not determine what are worthy human goals. Ethical decisions in uncharted areas require that scientific capabilities be understood and used by persons and communities sensitive to their own deepest convictions about human nature and destiny. There is no sound ethical judgment in these matters independent of scientific knowledge, but science does not itself prescribe the good.

Throughout this document we shall see many examples of the interaction of science and ethics. Responsible ethical decision-making will require the most accurate knowledge of new scientific possibilities, but will still have to ask which possibilities are humanly desirable. Such decision-making will need to measure risks with maximum precision, then will still have to decide what risks are morally justifiable. Some decisions require weighing the importance of personal freedom and of social goals or of immediate advantages and long-term consequences; again, scientific evidence contributes to a mature decision without fully answering age-old questions. When we come to ask which diseased lives are or are not worth living, we need the most rigorous scientific knowledge about diseases, but we must still ask what we mean by human life. When we try to decide whether foetal life at various stages has an inviolable human dignity, scientific data about foetal development will bear upon the answer, even though science alone cannot define human dignity.

As an example, we can take the effect of a given gene that may be harmful in one respect but beneficial in another, or harmful in some environments and beneficial in others. For example, the condition of glucose-6-phosphate dehydrogenase deficiency produces harmful results when the individual consumes fava beans or takes certain drugs, but it also confers increased resistance to malaria. Scientific judgment about such effects, even though incomplete, is indispensable for undersanding the case. Any moral judgment requires the best scientific information available. But after consideration of such information, judgments about harm and benefits are ultimately moral judgments.

As another example, consider the element of risk in the new procedure for prenatal diagnosis. At present the most effective method of intra-uterine diagnosis is amniocentesis, which involves withdrawal of some fluid from the amniotic sac within the uterus and the examination of the fluid and the foetal cells floating in it. Other techniques include foetoscopy and intrauterine photography, use of ultra-sound devices, and the highly experimental withdrawal of small blood samples from the foetus. In every case the risks of the procedure to foetus and to mother—a technical judgment—bear upon the ethical judgment of what human risks are justifiable for the sake of chosen human goals. The risks of amniocentesis appear to be small, but are not fully known. When amniocentesis is followed by abortion, there are additional physiological and psychological risks to the mother. Further experience may give more accurate knowledge of the risks and may reduce them. In any case, the reckoning of the risks will enter into the ethical judgment but will not entirely determine it. There is, after all, no life without risk, but some risks are rash and irresponsible. No diagnosis is completely reliable. We see a moral responsibility for medical institutions offering amniocentesis and consequent abortion to verify *prenatal* diagnoses after the abortion, as a contribution to more accurate diagnosis. A more detailed discussion of this example is given in section 2.

Another example is the relation of present benefit to future harm. Amniocentesis and selective abortion enable parents to avoid having children with defects that are diagnosable prenatally; but if the parents have another child in place of the one aborted, such a child, although not handicapped itself, may carry the detrimental genes and so increase the load of these genes in the population and perhaps build up trouble for future generations, for example haemophilia, muscular dystrophy and translocation Down's syndrome (*see* glossary). On the other hand, future generations may discover cures for present ailments. The estimate of present and future gains and harms is a scientific estimate, uncertain and always subject to revision. The weighing of present versus future values is an ethical issue.

The relationship between scientific advances and ethics also raises issues about medical decision-making, since physicians sometimes limit the availability of new techniques for reasons which they regard as scientific, but which actually belong to the sphere of values. For example, in some medical centres amniocentesis has been made conditional upon the woman's promising in advance to undergo an abortion should an affected foetus be diagnosed. The requirement of such a promise imposes a heavy burden on parental decision-making and excludes from the benefits of amniocentesis those patients who are uncertain about or presently opposed to abortion. Furthermore, a decision prior to diagnosis would be neither fully informed nor legally enforceable. On the other hand, amniocentesis is costly in its use of medical resources and entails risks (not yet fully defined) of morbidity and mortality for the mother and foetus; thus it cannot be undertaken lightly or solely for the sake of curiosity. After considering the costs and risks, parents may nevertheless decide to undertake amniocentesis without planning an abortion, so as to prepare themselves and their families for the birth of an affected child or to eliminate anxiety (which may even entail thoughts of an abortion) through a diagnosis that the foetus is unaffected by the condition for which the test was conducted.

These examples illustrate that neither Christians nor humanists can meet the future on the basis of past authoritative answers, that humane decisions require expert scientific knowledge, but that scientific knowledge does not itself constitute moral wisdom or sensitivity to human values.

2. **Foetal diagnosis and selective abortion** [1]

We turn to the investigation of one process made possible by recent genetic and medical discoveries. Some foetal abnormalities lead to spontaneous abortions, which prevent defective foetuses from developing to birth. However, other foetal abnormalities do not lead to spontaneous abortions. It has now become possible to diagnose some of these foetal defects and deliberately induce abortions. The ethical validity of such action is the question at issue.

a. *Criteria for responsible decisions*

In reaching a decision about foetal diagnosis and possible termination of pregnancy, a wide spectrum of genetic disorders has to be considered, ranging from cases so severe as to be incompatible with life to those which have only trivial effects. Therefore a number of criteria concerning the outlook for the prospective child must be taken into account.

The major criterion is obviously the severity of the abnormality in question. Other criteria are the availability of effective treatment and the welfare of family and society.

There are some genetic disorders which produce gross limitation of mental development, severe physical defects and marked curtailment of life. Tay-Sachs disease, for example, leads to mental degeneration, blindness and death in early childhood. Similarly in the Lesch-Nyhan

---

[1] In discussing the issue of foetal diagnosis and selective abortion, we are not taking up the more general issues of abortion. The judgments that apply in the one case do not necessarily apply in the other. Just as the arguments that support abortion for genetic reasons do not necessarily imply support for freely available abortion, so the legal availability of abortion does not morally justify selective abortion in the absence of adequate criteria.

syndrome, death occurs in most cases after a short life marked by spasticity and severe mental retardation, though there are a few known cases alive today as adolescents and young adults who are doing quite well on therapy. More common than either of these diseases is thalassemia major (Cooley's anaemia) which is frequently fatal before puberty. These disorders represent not only a major burden to family and society, but also, and most important of all, a short and humanly unfulfilling existence for the affected child.

In contrast there are many genetic abnormalities which have slight effect on the life style of the individual concerned, either because they produce few or no harmful effects or because they can be successfully managed medically with minimum difficulty and expense. Examples are myopia, colour blindness, achondroplastic (circus) dwarfism, gout (when treated) and glucose-6-phosphate dehydrogenase deficiency.

Between these two extremes lies a large range of genetic disorders where the appropriate decision as to the application of foetal diagnosis and abortion may be much less clear cut. Diseases such as phenylketonuria and galactosemia, which are medically manageable, at least partially, fall into this group. Down's syndrome, commonly called mongolism, provides still another type of situation: although the individual is at best unable to become entirely self-reliant, he nevertheless often has a happy disposition, freely giving and receiving affection though the majority tend to end their lives in an institution.

The effects of some genetic aberrations are as yet unclear. The XYY chromosomal constitution, for example, has been reported to be correlated with aggressiveness and even with criminal tendencies. Evidence for this association has been overemphasized and it is now apparent that only a small proportion of XYY males exhibit violent and dangerous behaviour. This case indicates that manifestation of a genetic abnormality in terms of anti-social behaviour may be dependent upon a particular social context.

It would be theoretically possible to construct a spectrum of genetic disorders, ranging from those most destructive of meaningful human life to those least threatening. At the one end would be those that convince some parents that they have not only a right but even a moral duty to seek abortion. At the other end would be those that are hard to justify ethically as grounds for abortion. In between would be the many, more problematic cases. Actually no precise spectrum can be made—for two reasons. First, information about and treatment of diseases change, with the result that the place of many genetic disorders on the spectrum changes. Second, because genetic disorders are always related to physical and human environments, the destructive threat of such disorders varies in different parts of the world and even in different families. For these reasons, and also because of varying moral convictions in different societies and families, we cannot catalogue the range of genetic disorders in relation to indications for foetal diagnosis and selective abortion.

We can say that a decision for foetal diagnosis and abortion is a weighty decision, as the foetus, although still dependent, has a potential existence as an independent human being,[2] excepting those cases such as anencephaly where the foetus may grow to term but cannot survive after separation from the uterus. The decision to deprive it of that potentiality depends on a conclusion that the detriments resulting from its birth outweigh the benefits.

Criteria that deserve to be employed by parents in reaching a decision include the following:

- The severity of the genetic disorder and its effect on the possibility of a meaningful life; or the probability of death, that is if death in infancy is certain some parents will prefer that to abortion;
- The physical, emotional and economic impact on family (parents and other children) and society;
- The availability of adequate medical management and of special educational and other facilities;
- The reliability of diagnosis and the predictability of the expression of the genetic disorder involved, both in degree and variability in manifestation of symptoms;
- The recognition that an individual genetically defective in one respect may be superior in others, and in fact may compensate (or even over-compensate) for his defect by development of other abilities or talents;
- The increase in the load of detrimental genes in the population that may result from the reproduction of carriers of genetic diseases.

b. *The roles of parents and professionals*

Decision-making about foetal diagnosis and abortion is difficult not only because it involves complicated and varied facts, as just described, but especially because it raises questions of life and death, health and suffering. As such it is a deeply personal decision, involving not only rational factors but also profound feelings, sensitivities, the self-awareness of husband and wife, and their mutual relationship.

---

[2] An abortion following amniocentesis usually comes at about the 18th to 20th week of foetal development. This is obligated by the nature of the procedures and the time taken to culture the fluid before a diagnosis can be made.

The choice to undertake foetal diagnosis or abortion, like all difficult decisions, must ultimately be made by individuals guided by their understanding of the facts and by their conscience; decision-making on these subjects is best governed, we believe, by the principle of responsible parenthood, that is, by placing the decision in the hands of the prospective parents to be exercised by them after a careful consideration of a number of factors. Their choice should, of course, be informed by expert advice from a physician competent in genetic counselling or other genetic counsellor; and in addition, according to their wishes, by consultation with their spiritual counsellors, family and friends. Furthermore it is not fair that the burden of weighing the issues should be borne by parents and counsellors alone: governments should also take the responsibility of investigating the relevant ethical and social issues and provide a supportive background of information. (See 4.d. and 5.) However, as with other decisions involving the family and child-rearing, the parents must remain the principal decision-makers.

A genetic counsellor must be sensitive to the great dangers of misunderstanding and confusion which arise in this emotionally charged area. It is also important that the parents receive psychological and spiritual support as required, to help them understand the choices open to them and to provide them with a context into which to fit the dictates of their own conscience. This context of decision may take the form of religious principles and traditions, a community consensus expressed through group decisions or laws, or in some instances restrictions formally imposed by the state.

c. *Priorities and costs*

The subject of foetal diagnosis and consequent abortion requires some discussion of priorities and costs. A more ethically concerned world would allot more resources to medical care, less resources to destructive and wasteful activities. Justice calls for major re-assignments of priorities. But in any foreseeable world no more than limited resources will be available for immense human needs. (*See also* 6.)

At present foetal diagnosis is available only on a limited basis, even in countries with advanced programmes. In most developing countries it is hardly available at all. The procedure is expensive, both in financial terms and in terms of staff and facilities needed; and it is likely to continue to be so, although some cost reductions are to be expected. A decision to make it more widely available depends on the judgment that its value ranks in priority with other urgent medical and social needs. On the other hand, the calculation of costs and priorities cannot ignore the costs of maintaining persons with genetic defects that could be detected by foetal diagnosis.

In many societies even the discussion of this possibility may appear as one more example of the widening gap between societies with high technology and the rest of the world. Hence any ethical decisions on this subject must take place in the context of the wide injustices that prevail in this world.

3. Genetic correction

Genetic correction refers to the alleviation of genetic defects. In the past this has largely involved the alleviation of symptoms in children and adults. New methods are now being developed to correct the defects prenatally.

Ordinary medicine proceeds with growing knowledge from a treatment of mere symptoms to various stages in the treatment of the cause. In the case of genetic disease the ultimate cause is a defective gene or genes. The role of the gene is to control the production of a specific kind of protein. For example, most of us have genes that control the production of normal haemoglobin in our red blood cells. But in some individuals one or more of these genes may be defective and an abnormal haemoglobin is produced, and consequently these persons suffer from anaemia. Or some genes may control the production of enzymes needed to permit normal mental development. The alteration of such genes is the cause, for example, of the mental retardation in phenylketonuria. Treatment may act at the level of the protein (for example, supplying insulin to a diabetic) or in the future by attempting to replace the defective gene with a normal gene. In principle there is no ethical difference between treatment at the level of the gene and treatment at the level of the symptoms as in ordinary medicine. The biochemical treatment moves from euphenics (changing the phenotype) to eugenics (changing the genotype). The treatment is no less biochemical. However, it does raise a number of ethical questions:

(1) A virus might be used as a carrier of the normal gene needed to replace the defective gene. This procedure is similar to existing procedures of inoculation with a virus to prevent smallpox or poliomyelitis. The development and use of inoculation has involved and still presents some risks which are ethically acceptable to most citizens because the benefits to the population greatly exceed the harm. **In the use of a virus as a carrier of a normal gene to replace a defective gene (when this becomes possible), the same attitude as is now acceptable for inoculation is applicable.**

(2) One new method for the alleviation of genetic disease is already practised. When the male parent is known to carry a defective gene causing a serious condition, artificial insemination using semen from a donor (AID) is sometimes employed. Some of us consider the use

of AID for this purpose as ethically acceptable provided the legitimate status of the offspring can be guaranteed, and laws should be modified, if necessary, to meet this situation. Those who advocated AID further believe that the source of the reproductive cell is far less important than the love, care and nurture of children, which they consider to be the essential element of parenthood. Others understand the Christian principle of the nonseparability of the marriage bond and the act of procreation as excluding any use of AID as morally unacceptable. Still others, who struggle with the moral uncertainties involved, may resort to AID only with some sense of guilt. **We recommend that Christians of different traditions be brought together by the WCC to give further careful thought to these issues.**

(3) Another method of averting the birth of children with genetic disease when the female is the carrier of a debilitating gene would be to donate to the woman an unfertilized egg which then can be fertilized in the normal way by the male parent. This method has obvious similarities to artificial insemination. It carries with it the same diversity of ethical judgments. **We recommend that Christians of different traditions be brought together by the WCC to give further careful thought to these issues.**

(4) A future possibility, when both parents carry the same defective gene as in the case of many recessive diseases, is the implantation of an early embryo derived from donors free of the defective gene. Such embryos will have to be produced by artificial fertilization in the laboratory. This method called prenatal adoption is not yet perfected. It would be a combination of the two preceding methods and is similar to post-natal adoption itself. Most people can see no basic ethical differences between this possible practice and the two preceding ones. Some persons on the other hand, having reluctantly accepted AID, feel that prenatal adoption means taking further steps in a very doubtful direction, and do not approve of it. Those who have no ethical objections to the methods referred to in (2), (3) and (4) above, argue further that because there are no children for adoption in many countries, these last three procedures are the only way whereby certain parents can have healthy children and avoid either childless families or the necessity of considering abortion of their natural foetuses which are defective. Moreover, they believe that the experience of pregnancy and birth may itself help to prepare the couple for the responsibilities of parenthood. **We recommend that Christians of different traditions be brought together by the WCC to give further careful thought to these issues.**

(5) Experimental studies on human embryos. The human egg when shed from the ovary is smaller than a pin-head. It remains approximately this size for the first five days after fertilization and during its early development as a tiny ball of cells, until the time of implantation into the uterus. Much information of value to prenatal health will be gained from studying these early stages of development, including the origin of several genetic disorders and the possibility of new forms of treatment. The organs begin to form in the foetus some thirty days after fertilization, and grow during succeeding days until the foetus has recognizable but rudimentary head, body and limbs. **The question of the acquisition of rights by embryos and foetuses (in these and later stages of their development) urgently requires discussion and interpretation.**

Medical information of considerable value could also be gained from the application of drugs and other agents to human embryos growing in culture, or to aborted foetuses. Such information could reveal how chromosomal abnormalities arise such as that which causes Down's syndrome. This might lead to means of averting genetic disease in the foetus.

We see no objection to the use of tissues from foetuses after death. However, the use of living foetuses presents issues which we are unable to agree on at this stage. There are some who are opposed on the grounds of the sacredness of human life at all stages. There are others who are concerned about inflicting pain or suffering on a possibly sensitive human foetus, and the possible dangers of misuse in obtaining foetuses. Others see no objection because these foetuses are doomed to die in any case and their use could benefit mankind, provided that (a) the foetus has not reached the stage of viability independent of the mother, which stage would need to be reassessed from time to time, and (b) these procedures are strictly supervised.

The deliberate culture of human embryos in order to use and destroy them for experimental purposes raises additional questions concerning the possible abuse of such procedures. We are unable to agree as to the ethical acceptability of such procedures. We understand that such experiments are not intended to be against human life but are undertaken as a means of scientific investigation in favour of greater knowledge of the genetic threats to human life. However, some believe that such experiments in themselves are ethically wrong. Others feel that the dangers of abuse outweigh the possible gains. Still others feel that the potential for good outweighs the danger of possible abuse. **We therefore advocate further study of the meaning of such scientific experiments** in. relation to the desire to maintain respect for human life in this special context.

4. Genetic counselling

In a broad sense we can consider genetic counselling to consist of at least two major components; education of the public and personal counselling. Technically the World Health Organization refers to the first as 'health education' and the second more specifically as 'genetic counselling'.

The most efficient way to deal with the need for public education is through a large-scale dissemination of information, using all available media, about genetic problems of general significance and about inherited conditions of significance to specific groups of people. This approach should help to promote a climate of opinion in which persons found to be carriers of mutant or unusual genes or affected with the disorders in question are least likely to be stigmatized or rejected by the larger community. If such education is presented in the context of community health (curative services, preventive medicine, family planning and health education), then the stigma now attached to hereditary diseases will probably be reduced, and people will be encouraged to seek professional advice.

The personal aspect of genetic counselling takes up the specific concerns of individuals, that is the medical, psychological, financial, social and ethical problems relating to the condition in question. Relevant information that may already have been presented in the educational programme will be reinforced, expanded and related to the individual life situation.

Genetic counselling, in its general education dimension, aims to inform, but can also appropriately influence attitudes and decisions. It is important therefore that the churches, in their teaching role, take an interest in seeing that genetic information is disseminated in a manner beneficial to humanity as a whole, while guarding the best interests of persons.

Genetic counselling, in its personal dimension, aims to help individuals or families to arrive at informed decisions without inappropriate influence. Here too the churches have an interest because of their concern for the welfare of persons. The present document devotes more space to this personal dimension of counselling which is the field of competence of the panel. However, we do not thereby imply that the general education dimension of counselling is less important.

a. *Persons deserving counselling*

There are at least four distinct groups of people for whom genetic counselling is of value:

(1) About half the people who visit counsellors are parents of off-spring which are malformed or have other damage of unknown origin in which genes may or may not play a part. The parents want to know whether the disorder is likely to occur in subsequent children and what measures they can take to care for the child they already have.

(2) Less frequently, an adult finds himself affected with a disorder, for example, Huntington's chorea, porphyria, diabetes, deafness, epilepsy, and wants to know whether the problem is of genetic origin and whether it is likely to occur in his or her children.

(3) Sometimes prospective parents know of relatives affected with an inherited disorder and wish to know more about the disease and the likelihood of its occurrence in themselves and/or their children. Cousins contemplating marriage form a special group of some import-ance because risks have invariably been overemphasized.

(4) More recently, the advent of large-scale genetic testing pro-grammes or mass genetic screening programmes has brought for coun-selling persons found to be carriers of genes determining dominant or recessively inherited diseases, for example sickle cell anaemia, porphyria, or Tay-Sachs disease. They want information about the disease, the way it is inherited, and the chance of their having affected children.

In the latter two groups much needless anxiety may arise where there is little or no chance that an inherited condition will occur. Much of this anxiety can be prevented by effective educational programmes. Where genetically determined defects occur, parents often experience significant feelings of guilt and self-depreciation. Dissemination of gene-tic information is always emotion-laden. Provisions should be made in counselling for recognition and management of psychological needs. Couples may try to blame one another for the birth of the abnormal child, and this can create serious disruption within the marriage. Such problems may spring from individual differences in emotional make-up or may reflect the nature of the marital relationship. Nevertheless, these difficulties can be reduced or alleviated by an effective educational pro-gramme combined with adequate psychological services.

b. *Objectives of counselling*

The objectives of any genetic counselling programme will usually pre-determine the spirit in which it is carried out and will include all factors involved—psychological, social and ethical. In the medical or health care setting, counselling should be patient or client-oriented. The counsellor has a responsibility to keep the welfare of the person seeking counsel as his primary aim; if this is not the case, this should be made clear to the client in advance. Counselling can help in:

(1) Marriage decisions: by providing a setting and information that will help young people make informed decisions in choosing marriage partners.

(2) Reproductive decisions: by providing information to individuals and couples that will help them make informed decisions about their future reproduction; to inform parents who already have an affected child about the risks that this as well as other inherited disorders may recur in succeeding children; to inform persons who are in doubt as to whether their own disease or handicap may be passed on to their children.

(3) Family and social implications: by assisting parents to plan for the future care of an affected child, and to help them in the acceptance of this child into their lives, their family and the community.

(4) In pregnancy: by informing pregnant women actively seeking advice about the possible risks of specific inherited or genetically determined diseases, for example older women (over thirty-eight years) who may have chromosomal disorders in the foetus diagnosable *in utero*.

(5) To remove guilt and forms of incrimination of self or spouse by providing correct information and comprehensive explanation.

c. *Principles of genetic counselling*

Genetic counselling can take many forms, but patient-oriented counselling achieves its objectives by adhering to the following essential principles:

(1) All forms of genetic counselling must be based on an accurate diagnosis of the disorder in question. The counsellor must be certain not only that he is dealing with an inherited condition, but that the mode of inheritance has been correctly determined (patients with the same or similar sets of abnormalities may have inherited them via different genetic mechanisms). The counsellor need not be a physician, but since correct diagnosis is so essential to proper genetic counselling, it is best carried out in a medical setting in association with or under the direction of a competent physician, except for the simplest and most obvious inherited conditions. Ideally, genetic counselling should be an integral part of the health care of the society, available to everyone on request. The physician or other competently trained health worker should be equipped to do the counselling. Since genetic counselling is a relatively recent addition to the spectrum of health services, all genetic counsellors will require some level of specialized training. Wherever feasible, counselling should take place in a setting where special diagnostic evaluation or therapeutic measures can be undertaken. Nevertheless, in developing countries, or areas with a serious shortage of physicians,

and where diagnostic evaluation and therapeutic measures may be at a minimum, all categories of health workers may require enough familiarity with genetic problems to allow for appropriate professional investigation and counselling.

(2) Information relevant to the condition in question should be clearly and simply presented. Areas where there is uncertainty or where information is missing should be highlighted. Information should be presented without bias.

(3) Counselling involves an implicit contract between counsellor and counselee in which the interest of the counselee in making his or her own informed decision is basic. Such an informed decision requires a full consideration of the interests of the individual, the family, the society and future generations. Since the counsellor is in a unique position where he could unconsciously direct the counselee to make decisions which were not his or her own, the counsellor's aim must be to present all relevant facts to the counselee. The counsellor must strive to avoid promoting his personal views of any of the issues—individual, familiar or social—unless they are clearly identified as such.

(4) The counsellor and related professionals should support the counselee in facing the social and emotional factors involved in the decision-making process.

(5) The counselling process should be kept strictly confidential. When the diagnosis indicates that relatives of the counselee are also at risk of serious genetic illness, the counsellor should seek the counselee's permission to contact the relatives through their physician, as a normal part of a person's responsibilities to his fellows.

(6) Counsellors should be persons who are intelligent, sensitive, concerned, highly motivated, able to relate to different types of people and whose primary concern is for the welfare and rights of the counselee. Properly trained clergymen could make a valuable contribution in this role; they would be especially valuable in follow-up work to ascertain whether counselled persons understand the information (especially the risk estimates) which has been given to them.

d. *An approach to informed decision-making*
The counsellor, working with parents or prospective parents, can help them understand the nature and severity of genetic disorders. The variety of handicaps either partly or wholly genetic in origin is enormous. However, independently of exact etiology or mechanism, most of the handicaps present themselves to the family and the counsellor as one of the following clinical pictures and problems:
• Children with a progressively fatal degenerative disease.

- Children who are at risk to a diseased condition with varying expressions which can range from trivial to catastrophic.
- Severely retarded children, needing in most cases full institutionalization.
- Mildly retarded children, therefore educable in special schools.
- Children needing constant and diligent care so as not to become retarded (for example suffering from phenylketonuria or galactosemia).
- Children with motor handicaps, but mentally normal or nearly normal (all the varieties of cerebral palsy).
- Children needing very specialized surgical and medical care for the correction of their abnormalities and who will still remain handicapped (for example major abnormalities of the central nervous system such as hydrocephaly).
- Children kept in reasonable health with constant medical care but with a greatly reduced chance at present of survival beyond puberty. Here the main example is thalassemia major (Cooley's anaemia), perhaps the most important genetic problem in some countries.
- Persons with conditions not apparent in childhood but becoming manifest in adulthood, for example Huntington's chorea.

In addition to understanding the nature and severity of genetic disorders, persons faced with decisions will want to know the statistical severity of the risk that a future child may have a genetically determined disease. The magnitude of the risk varies considerably from one condition to the other (*see also* 4.c.). For example, there is a 100 per cent risk that the baby born to a parent carrying a specific chromosome aberration will be affected with Down's syndrome. The risk in other cases may be less; for example, the risk is 2 to 10 per cent for the newborn of a parent carrying a particular chromosomal translocation in balanced form of having the same translocation in unbalanced form and so being affected also by Down's syndrome. In Tay-Sachs disease, where both parents are carriers, there is a 25 per cent chance in each pregnancy of the child being affected.

Factors that need to be taken into account when making a decision are:
- Biomedical factors of the condition and its possible impact on the family, including care required and probable outcome.
- Financial implications.
- Genetic factors, including the hereditary mechanism and risk of occurrence or recurrence. (Special effort should be made to ensure understanding that genetic prediction is based on probability and not on certainty.)

- Potential social problems or conflicts, including effects on the gene pool (*see* 5.).
- Possible emotional and psychological repercussions.
- Consideration of all available reproductive options.
- Resolution of ethical or moral conflicts.
- Potential for cure or partial cure; it is important to convey hope when such is a reasonable prospect.

e. *Some elements of Christian ethics which have direct application to the genetic counselling situation*

In genetic counselling, there is a particular need for the recognition on the part of all involved of the place of their personal conscience in making a moral decision. The conscience of the person seeking counsel, informed by the teachings of his church and acting in terms not only of his own interests but also in terms of his relationship with other persons and with God, is the practical norm of moral decision.

The counsellor should respect completely the beliefs, values, attitudes, freedom and conscience of the client, actively helping him at the same time to see the options and to reflect on the possible consequences of his decision.

With regard to decisions resulting from genetic counselling, the church should reflect the care and the compassion of God for those who are in situations where whatever is decided is foreseen to have distressing consequences. When persons are confronted with dilemmas in which none of the possible choices is free from moral conflict, or have acted contrary to the teachings of the church, the church should mirror God's compassionate acceptance and understanding of humanity.

Christian concern, especially for the troubled, the suffering, the poor, the weak and the helpless, as well as for the promotion of total health for all people, should be shown by the counsellor and communicated to the person seeking counsel (*see* 1.b.).

The very difficult question of how to reconcile care and respect for genetically handicapped individuals, with prevention of more such individuals being born, can rarely be coped with fruitfully except in the context of a soundly based and well worked-out world-view, in which all dimensions of human life, including the spiritual one, are taken into account. The churches have here a special study, and their theologians should not only think these matters through and give direction; they should also learn to understand the experience of the genetically afflicted parents and of those who are directly concerned to help them, for that is how new insights are won.

f. *Recommendations*

On the basis of the foregoing considerations, we make the following recommendations on genetic counselling:

(1) Since the physician inevitably plays a leading role in genetic counselling, it is essential that medical students and other related health professions receive more comprehensive training in genetics than is now offered in most medical schools.

(2) Since correct diagnosis is so essential to proper genetic counselling, the latter is best carried out in association with or under the direction of a competent physician, except for the simplest and most obvious inherited conditions.

(3) Representatives of the churches, physicians and geneticists should together regularly prepare material suitable for general dissemination about progress in human genetics and the new ethical problems this progress may entail.

(4) Because of the need for continuing support over varying periods of time, the genetic counsellor should, where possible, be in a position to enlist the aid of a team of helpers. Among these, properly trained church personnel have a very significant place.

(5) It is important that long-term follow-up be undertaken of families who have received genetic counselling, both for their own benefit and also to extend our knowledge in this comparatively new field.

5. The changing genetic constitution of mankind

The reservoirs of genes in human populations are called 'gene pools'. Two fundamental facts must be understood about gene pools. First, every interbreeding population has a different genetic composition. The differences may be in frequencies of the various blood groups or other properties, or in the incidence of genes producing genetic anomalies of varying degrees of severity. Second, the content of the gene pool of any population is constantly undergoing change from generation to generation.

In the past this change occurred without conscious human intervention. Because of mutation, natural selection, migration and other evolutionary processes, certain genes would rise in frequency and others would fall in patterns which would differ in various populations. In particular, genes producing very severe genetic defects would be kept at a low incidence, if the individuals carrying them were unable to procreate. This phenomenon is, of course, still occurring for many genes in different populations. But two important considerations have newly arisen. First, the reduction and increased uniformity of family size which is being witnessed in many societies is rapidly reducing the margin on which natural selection can operate. Thus, when family size varied from zero to ten or more children, the more prolific families contributed more genes to the subsequent generation. But the more uniform the size of families the less will be the selection.

The second problem arises from the possibility that is or may soon be provided by the advances in biological science and biological technology for a deliberate manipulation of the gene pool. There are many avenues open for this purpose. Genetic correction, considered in a separate section of this report, is one. Genetic counselling, also considered in a separate section of this report, can lead to changes in reproductive patterns of carriers of specific genes, thereby affecting their frequencies. Prevention of reproduction by specific groups of individuals will also affect the gene pools.

In contrasting the effects of genetic correction and of genetic counselling on gene pools, we shall at the moment refer only to methods available now for correction of the phenotype, rather than the therapy of the gene itself, which may be possible in the future. Clearly, the correction of a genetic defect increases on the average the reproductive potential of its carrier. Hence, frequency of the gene causing the abnormality will climb. For instance, the invention of spectacles has no doubt increased the incidence of people with imperfect vision. This may be a trivial burden on society. But restoring normal reproductive fitness by therapy to such defects as diabetes and the very debilitating Tay-Sachs disease is another matter. It is true that when the disease is caused by a recessive gene, the rise in its frequency will be exceedingly slow. But in the case of a rare disease caused by a dominant gene, fully effective therapy will lead to a doubling of the incidence in the first generation.

If public education and counselling lead carriers of genetic defects to have no children, fewer children, or to resort to artificial insemination, or to prenatal or post-natal adoption, the frequency of undesirable genes may be reduced. Some have advocated with some logic that a person whose life has been saved by therapy might express their responsibility to the society which has given them life by foregoing the having of children and so not passing on the deleterious genes.

While the question of happiness of children or of parents is primarily a matter of individual concern, the burden of an increasing load of defective genes is a matter for society as well as individuals to consider.

6. **Decision-making by individuals and society**

We have earlier emphasized (4.b and 4.c) the importance of informed personal decisions, uncoerced by counsellors or government. We now point out that even the most freely made personal decisions take place in a social context. Public policies do, for better or worse, influence decisions; such policies therefore require attention.

As one example, cultural attitudes affect individuals and their decisions. In many societies, there is strong pressure to marry and have children because of the idea that full self-achievement can only be achieved by a person in that way. Such pressures should not prevent some men and women from remaining celibate and childless through voluntary choice. Society needs both dedicated parents and persons dedicated wholly to other forms of service and achievement.

As another example, educational opportunity and economic status affect the options available to people. For this reason it is important that medical men and others should educate the authorities in public health and the wider public in the problems of human genetics. Most genetic advice is sought after the child is born and therefore is usually too late. There should be counselling during the prenatal period and even before conception. The number of people who are aware of and use genetic counselling is too low; nine-tenths of those who seek counsel already have one defective child, and in the remainder there is some family indication of an inherited disease. Unfortunately, most of those who seek advice belong to the wealthier classes, and many in the poorer classes who urgently need advice cannot get it. Studies have shown that many who think they understand the problems of genetic disease do not fully appreciate the issues involved and do not know where to turn for better advice. Family doctors are often unable to help and can actually mislead.

To go a step further, there are situations in which society has a major stake, as it has long recognized in the case of contagious diseases. Decisions will be made at given times and places by whatever machinery is thought to be optimal. In the case of genetic disease such decision will not be easy. How serious must the defect (which may range from ragweed pollen allergy or myopia to lethal and horrifying diseases such as the Lesch-Nyhan syndrome) before any social action is undertaken? The precise line has to be arbitrary, but the issue is ambiguous. Similarly, how high should the incidence of a defect be permitted to rise, when it is costly to cure and therefore calls for mass therapeutic programmes which have to compete for priority in the distribution of a society's resources? Specific problems and their answers may be primarily the concern of particular societies, but development of some general ethical guidelines has some ecumenical urgency.

The mutual responsibilities of society and individual have to be re-evaluated in the face of these new ways of preventing misfortunes that previously were thought to be inevitable. **There is, in our view, a significant new task for the churches in all countries to help men and women to understand and discharge these responsibilities.**

Whatever should be done to correct genetic defects in individuals or in the population, there is a clear ethical demand that the people involved participate in policy decisions. Democratic procedures are admittedly very imperfect, but there are no better ways. The old question, 'Who controls the controller?', is an endlessly recurring one that can never be finally answered; nevertheless we have to try.

The procedures that we wish to recommend are as follows:

Hospital committees are needed to decide on how resources (of people, material, space, and so on) should be used for different patients and groups of patients. Such committees already exist in various forms in various places, and they have many other things to decide besides genetic questions. But now they must give attention to questions like these: Who can be given amniocentesis? How much time is to be spent on genetic counselling? What kinds of operation are permissible? In so far as such questions lie within the competence of the hospital itself, they should be decided by a team as widely representative as possible, including not only medical (and scientific) personnel on all levels but also geneticists and representatives of the patients (often their parents).

However, the vital decisions on social policy concerning genetics must generally be taken at the state or national level. **Where science has brought new possibilities of modifying the human genetic make-up, parliaments and governments should take the responsibility of looking into the relevant social and ethical issues, not leaving them entirely to the doctors, counsellors, parents or other people directly involved. It is not fair to let them bear this burden alone, and society does not expect this of them in other fields. Furthermore, governments should bear much, if not all, of the cost of care and treatment of the unfortunate victims of genetic disease and should support research on further advances in treatment.**

In some countries, preliminary committees are already looking into these questions and asking where new legislation may be necessary. What must be decided are answers to questions like these: What sort of experiments on humans and foetuses are legal and what are not? Should genetic counsellors be subject to professional regulations? What diseases with a genetic background are—in each particular country— serious enough to warrant a mass screening programme, involving perhaps amniocentesis and selective abortion? Should abortion in such cases ever be made compulsory? To what fields should more money be directed for new research, and what research should consequently get less money? Where must cost-benefit analyses be made of different public health programmes and measures? How far should governments go in putting the financial burden of caring for genetically handicapped children on the taxpayer other than the parents? Even the pinpointing of such questions is liable to raise violent objections of many kinds, but this does not make it any less necessary to start the debate.

It is quite reasonable to foresee that if committees, consisting of representatives of various professions and various interest groups, including the churches, are to be set up to consider the above questions, the result may be an inhibiting of certain kinds of research and the approval of only innocuous measures. This is a risk society always has to take. The chief benefit of such committees, at least in their initial stages, would probably be a general raising of consciousness among the general public. We need not only a spreading of factual information, which is always to the good, but also a heightened awareness of the moral issues involved and the necessity of taking deliberate thought on things that we have hitherto trusted nature to do for us, whether well or badly. We commend the establishment of such committees of a non-governmental nature as have already been set up.

Above the national level, there are international organizations, chiefly the World Health Organization (WHO) and the Council for International Organizations of the Medical Sciences (CIOMS). They have already touched on the subject. **We urge the WHO (if useful, in collaboration with UNESCO) to set up a committee of the kind advocated at the 1972 Paris meeting of CIOMS. This would put the experts on genetics all over the world in a position to explain to all nations what measures they think should be taken, globally, regionally or nationally, in order to channel the results of modern genetic insight into programmes acceptable to governments and peoples.**

The ways of using modern genetics to help afflicted populations will no doubt be different in different parts of the world. A global genetic programme is very far off. For some countries, these measures must have lower priority than for others. It must be made very clear that no country or group of countries should try to dictate its genetic policies to any other, whether under the guise of aid or otherwise. To many persons, the dangers are very real of abuse of genetic programmes in the name of ethics, science or the future of humanity.

7. Summary of recommendations

(1)   The principle of responsible parenthood requires that, whatever the help needed and given, specific decisions about foetal diagnosis and abortion must be made by the parents concerned.

(2) The criteria presently applied in decisions about inoculation will be adequate for the eventual possibility of replacing defective genes by means of a virus.

(3) Further study should be encouraged, by the World Council of Churches and other ecumenical agencies, of the ethical issues arising out of the use for genetic correction of artificial insemination (AID), ova donation and prenatal adoption.

(4) The experimental study of human embryos raises urgent questions about the rights of embryos and foetuses.

(5) Further study is necessary of what it means to maintain respect for human life in relation to scientific experiments involving the culture of human embryos.

(6) More comprehensive training in genetics needs to be given to medical students and others in the health professions.

(7) Genetic counselling is best carried out in close association with a competent physician.

(8) Material about progress in genetic research and the ethical issues this may entail should regularly be prepared by church representatives, physicians and geneticists, working together, for general education of the public.

(9) Genetic counsellors need to be able to draw on the services of a team of helpers, in which properly trained church persons can have a significant place.

(10) Long-term follow-up should be arranged in the case of families who have received genetic counselling.

(11) The allocation of resources between different patients and groups of patients needs to be decided by appropriately constituted hospital committees.

(12) The burden of genetic decisions cannot be left entirely to doctors, counsellors and parents but must be shared, by appropriate studies and financial grants, by governments.

(13) We urge the World Health Organization to establish a committee which could explain to governments and peoples what measures need to be taken at different levels in order to channel the results of genetic research into appropriate programmes.

Glossary

AID: Artificial insemination by donor. Fertilization of the ovum within the woman's body by artificial introduction into the vagina of semen from a donor other than the woman's husband. The child resulting from the process receives half its inheritance from the mother, half from the donor.

Amniocentesis: A method of prenatal diagnosis. A needle is used to withdraw some fluid from the amniotic sac within the uterus of the pregnant woman. The fluid and foetal cells floating in it can then be examined, usually after growth in a culture. By this method some genetic disorders can be diagnosed prior to birth.

Chromosomal translocation: The attachment of a portion of one chromosome to another, for example, as in translocation Down's syndrome.

Chromosome: The structure in the cell that carries the genetical material deoxyribonucleic acid (DNA) that constitutes the genes. There are normally forty-six in each human cell.

Cystic fibrosis: A hereditary disease characterized by malfunctioning of the pancreas and glands responsible for secretion of mucus. It is most frequent among people of North European descent.

Dominant: In genetics, an inherited trait which appears in the physical make-up of the person bearing the gene for that trait. *See* recessive.

Down's syndrome: Sometimes called mongolism. A condition resulting from chromosomal abnormality. It involves mental retardation (moderate or severe) and certain characteristic physical features. There are two forms: trisomy, which is caused by a chromosome added to chromosome no. 21, and chromosomal translocation. *See above.*

Eugenics: (good genotype) The improvement of the genetical constitution of man. Negative eugenics is the restriction of reproduction of those individuals whose progeny might be genetically defective. Positive eugenics is the encouragement of production of progeny using sex cells of parents of 'desirable' genetical constitution.

Euphenics: (good phenotype) Therapy that counteracts the deleterious effects of disease, for example, the use of insulin in diabetes.

Foetoscopy: A technique for visual observation of the foetus within the uterus.

Galactosemia: A hereditary disease, which unless treated in the first month of life, results in mental retardation and lesions of various organs because the child is unable to utilize galactose effectively.

Genotype: The genetic constitution of the person. *See* phenotype.

Gene: The basic unit of heredity. It consists of deoxyribonucleic acid (DNA). The chromosome is the carrier of the genes.

Gene pool: The reservoir of genes in a population, i.e. the sum total of all the genes in all individuals in the population.

Haemophilia: A hereditary disorder transmitted by symptomless females, characterized by a tendency to uncontrollable bleeding following injury.

Huntington's chorea: A hereditary disease which develops in mid-life, resulting in mental deterioration and uncontrollable movements of the limbs.

Hydrocephaly: A hereditary disorder resulting in enlargement of the head due to accumulation of cerebrospinal fluid in internal spaces of the brain and sometimes associated mental retardation, only rarely inherited.

Intra-uterine photography: A recently developed technique comparable to foetoscopy, but involving the photography (rather than simply the observation) of the foetus within the uterus.

Lesch-Nyhan syndrome: A hereditary disease, usually causing death in childhood.

Muscular dystrophy: A hereditary disease producing muscle cell destruction and hence muscle weakness especially in the limbs and spinal muscles.

Phenotype: The physical constitution of the individual, as distinguished from the genetic constitution or genotype.

Phenylketonuria (PKU): A genetic disorder due to an enzyme deficiency, with severe mental deficiency unless treated early in infancy.

Porphyria: A hereditary disease in which excessive amounts of porphyrin are excreted with associated pain and nervous symptoms.

Recessive: An inherited trait that does not appear in the parent who is a 'carrier' of it, but which may appear in the child if transmitted by both parents. See dominant.

Sex-linked diseases: Those diseases which are due to genes on the X-chromosome and usually affect only males, for example, haemophilia, Lesch-Nyhan syndrome, muscular dystrophy.

Sickle cell anaemia: A genetically caused anaemia, affecting principally people of African origin.

Tay-Sachs disease: A hereditary disease involving neurological degeneration, blindness and death in early childhood. Occurs almost exclusively among people of Ashkenaz-Jewish descent.

Thalassemia major, or Cooley's anaemia: A hereditary blood disease often fatal before puberty. It is commonest amongst Mediterranean peoples.

XYY Syndrome: A chromosomal abnormality in which the male has an extra Y chromosome, the effects of which are incompletely known.

Participants

Chairman
Prof. Charles Birch
Challis Professor of Biology, University of Sydney, Sydney, Australia

Human geneticists
Dr F. I. D. Konotey-Ahulu
Department of Medicine and Therapeutics, Clinical Hereditary Erythrocytopathy Research, Korle Bu Teaching Hospital, Ghana
Prof. I. Michael Lerner
Professor of Genetics, University of California, Berkeley, Calif., USA
Dr E. Matsunaga
Head of Department of Human Genetics, National Institute of Genetics, Misima, Japan
Prof. Angelo Serra, s.j.
Director, Institute of Human Genetics, Faculty of Medicine and Surgery, Catholic University of the Sacred Heart, Rome, Italy
Prof. Dr H. Ursprung
President, Swiss Federal Institute of Technology, Zurich, Switzerland

Molecular and reproductive biologists
Dr R. G. Edwards
Department of Physiology, University of Cambridge, Cambridge, England
Prof. Bentley Glass
Department of Cellular and Comparative Biology, State University of New York, Stony Brook, New York, USA
Dr Barbara Sanford
Microbiologist, Harvard University School of Public Health, Cambridge, Mass., USA

Obstetricians, medical geneticists and paediatricians
Dr A. E. Boyo
Professor and Head of Department of Pathology, College of Medicine, University of Lagos, Nigeria
Prof. Spyros Doxiadis
Institute of Child Health, Athens, Greece
Dr T. Kajii
Laboratory of Embryology and Cytogenetics, University Clinic of Gynaecology and Obstetrics, Geneva, Switzerland
Dr Robert Murray
Associate Professor of Paediatrics and Medicine, Howard University, Washington, DC, USA
Prof. Rolf Zetterström
St Göran's Children's Hospital, Stockholm, Sweden

Psychiatrist
Dr Miles F. Shore
New England Medical Center Hospital, Boston, Mass., USA

Medical and social research workers
Dr Katherine Elliott
Assistant Director, CIBA Foundation, London, England
Prof. Dr med. W. Tünte
Institute for Human Genetics, Münster, West Germany

Lawyers, legislators and others
Dr Kerstin Anér
Member of Parliament, Stockholm, Sweden
Prof. Alexander M. Capron
Assistant Professor of Law, University of Pennsylvania, Philadelphia, USA

Mr Bruce Hilton
  Editor, *Genetic Counseling,* Leonia,
  NJ, USA
Dr Rihito Kimura
  Lawyer on the Staff of the Ecu-
  menical Institute, Geneva, Switzer-
  land
Mr H. van Looy
  Director, Institute for Mentally
  Handicapped, Turnhout, Belgium
Mr Davidson Sommers
  Consultant to the World Bank,
  Washington, DC, USA
Theologians
Dr Günter Altner
  Professor of Theology and Bio-
  logical Sciences, Heidelberg, West
  Germany
Prof. André Dumas
  Theologian, Protestant Faculty,
  Paris, France
Fr Robert Faricy, s.j.
  Theological Faculty, Gregorian
  University, Vatican City

Dr Ellen Flesseman-van Leer
  Theologian, Netherlands
Prof. Roger Shinn
  Professor of Christian Ethics,
  Union Theological Seminary, New
  York, USA
Fr Paul Verghese
  Dean of the Syrian Orthodox Theo-
  logical Seminary, Kerala, India
Christian Medical Commission
Mrs Helen Gideon
  Medical doctor
Prof. Pieter Janssens
  Director, Institute of Tropical
  Medicine, Antwerp, Belgium
Sister Gilmary Simmons
  Medical doctor

Other WCC staff
Mr Paul Abrecht
  Executive Secretary, Department
  on Church and Society
Miss Frances Smith
  Press Officer

Index